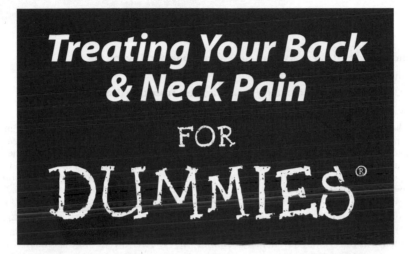

Treating Your Back & Neck Pain

FOR DUMMIES®

by Dr Loïc Burn, Michael S. Sinel, MD, and William W. Deardorff, PhD

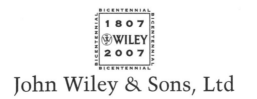

BICENTENNIAL
1807
WILEY
2007
BICENTENNIAL

John Wiley & Sons, Ltd

Treating Your Back & Neck Pain For Dummies®

Published by
John Wiley & Sons, Ltd
The Atrium
Southern Gate
Chichester
West Sussex
PO19 8SQ
England

E-mail (for orders and customer service enquires): cs-books@wiley.co.uk

Visit our Home Page on www.wiley.com

Wiley also publishes its books in a variety of electronic formats. Some content that appears in print may not be available in electronic books.

British Library Cataloguing in Publication Data: A catalogue record for this book is available from the British Library.

ISBN: 978-0-470-03599-3

Printed and bound in Great Britain by Bell and Bain Ltd, Glasgow

10 9 8 7 6 5 4 3 2 1

WILEY

About the Authors

Dr Loïc Burn is a specialist physician in the Department of Musculoskeletal Medicine, the Royal London Homeopathic Hospital, University College London Hospitals NHS Trust. He is a vice president of BackCare, past president of the International Federation for Manual Medicine, past president of the British Association of Manipulative Medicine, former member of the Executive Committee of the Scientific Section of the British League Against Rheumatism, former member of the Council of Management, medical adviser to BackCare, and editor of the professional supplement to Talkback, the magazine for BackCare members. He is an author of the Diploma of Primary Care Rheumatology offered by the University of Bath, former clinical tutor to the spinal module, and Chairman of the Education Committee of the Primary Care Rheumatology Society. Dr Burn is the author of six books, has edited two, and has appeared on national television and radio as a back specialist.

Michael Sinel, MD is a renowned back pain expert. He received his medical degree from the State University of New York Downstate and then completed a residency in physical medicine and rehabilitation at New York Hospital-Cornell University Medical Center. After serving as Director of Outpatient Physical Medicine at Cedar Sinai Medical Center, he became board-certified in both physical medicine and rehabilitation and pain management.

Dr Sinel is a co-founder of California Orthopedics and Rehabilitation (COR), a prestigious multi-specialty medical group in Beverly Hills, California. He is also an assistant clinical professor at UCLA Medical Center and attending physician with the UCLA Comprehensive Spine Center. He lectures regularly to various medical and lay audiences and is actively involved in clinical research of spinal disorders.

As a specialist in non-surgical approaches to spinal problems and pain management, Dr Sinel has made numerous national radio and television appearances and has been quoted in *The New York Times*, *Los Angeles Times*, and *Reader's Digest*.

William W. Deardorff, PhD, ABPP received his doctorate in clinical psychology with a special emphasis in health from Washington State University after completing an internship at the University of Washington Medical School. He then completed a post-doctoral fellowship in behavioural medicine at Kaiser Permanente Medical Center in Los Angeles.

Dr Deardorff is board-certified in clinical health psychology and specialises in the evaluation and treatment of psychological issues related to medical problems. He is a Fellow of the American Psychological Association and Past-President of the American Academy of Clinical Health Psychology. Dr Deardorff is in practice with California Orthopedic and Rehabilitation group in Beverly Hills, California. As an assistant clinical professor at the UCLA School of Medicine, he is active in teaching and research.

Dr Deardorff has published extensively in the area of health psychology. His previous patient guidebook, *Preparing for Surgery: A Mind-Body Approach to Enhance Healing and Recovery* won the Small Press Book Award in Health in 1998. He has made numerous national radio and television appearances, and has been quoted in a variety of general publications.

Authors' Acknowledgements

Loïc Burn: I would like to thank BackCare and in particular Nia Taylor, their Chief Executive for their help. I also thank my colleague Dr Adam Ward, with whom I have worked closely over the past decade, for his interest, support, and sage advice.

Michael Sinel: I want to thank my wife and my parents for their support and encouragement. I want to thank my first mentor, John Sarno, M.D., who taught me the strength of the mind-body connection, and my present and forever mentor and friend, Ted Goldstein, MD, who remains the premier 'spine doctor' in my eyes. Finally, I would like to thank my patients who will always be my true teachers.

William Deardorff: Aside from my family, I want to thank my close friends for their consistent support throughout the past year: Jeff and Kimberly Steinbach, Brian and Nicoli Tucker, Rick and Joanne Wilson, Ron and Gerri Day, and 'Uncle' Dr Allan F. Chino. I would also like to extend special thanks to Dr Theodore ('Teddy') Goldstein for his friendship, support, and professional practice style.

We would also like to thank the following for their contributions (listed in alphabetical order): Aaron Filler, MD; Mary Jo Ford, MD; Theodore Goldstein, MD; Stephen Hochschuler, MD; Patrick Johnson, MD; Fred Lerner, DC, PhD; Larry Payne, PhD; Joshua Prager, MD; John Reeves, II, PhD; Risa Sheppard; Stephen Sideroff, PhD; Jay Triano, DC, PhD; Steven Waldman, MD.

Publisher's Acknowledgements

We're proud of this book; please send us your comments through our Dummies online registration form located at www.dummies.com/register/.

Some of the people who helped bring this book to market include the following:

Acquisitions, Editorial, and Media Development

Project Editor: Rachael Chilvers

Content Editor: Steve Edwards

Development Editor: Colette Holden

Copyeditor: Andy Finch

Proofreader: Lesley Green

Technical Editor: Chris Murphy, www.physiouk.co.uk

Executive Editor: Jason Dunne

Executive Project Editor: Martin Tribe

Cover Photo: © Kaz Chiba/GettyImages

Cartoons: Ed McLachlan

Special Help: Jennifer Bingham and Zoë Wykes

Anniversary Logo Design: Richard J. Pacifico

Composition Services

Project Coordinator: Jennifer Theriot

Layout and Graphics: Lavonne Cook, Joyce Haughey, Stephanie D. Jumper, Laura Pence

Photos: Biofeedback: Robert Goldstein/ Science Photo Library

Proofreaders: Jessica Kramer, Susan Moritz

Indexer: Techbooks

Publishing and Editorial for Consumer Dummies

    Diane Graves Steele, Vice President and Publisher, Consumer Dummies

    Joyce Pepple, Acquisitions Director, Consumer Dummies

    Kristin A. Cocks, Product Development Director, Consumer Dummies

    Michael Spring, Vice President and Publisher, Travel

    Kelly Regan, Editorial Director, Travel

Publishing for Technology Dummies

    Andy Cummings, Vice President and Publisher, Dummies Technology/General User

Composition Services

    Gerry Fahey, Vice President of Production Services

    Debbie Stailey, Director of Composition Services

Contents at a Glance

Table of Contents

Introduction

'*O*h, my aching back!' If you've ever uttered these words more than a few times, this book's for you. Back and neck pain are very common problems. In fact, almost everyone experiences back or neck pain at some point in his or her life. Back and neck pain are closely linked. Up to 60 per cent of people with low back pain also report some neck symptoms.

We know how miserable back and neck pain can be: Many of our patients struggle with chronic back or neck pain, and others come to us searching for an end to pain that began after a car accident or other trauma. Several things can cause back and neck pain: This book suggests lots of remedies to manage – and conquer – these frustrating conditions.

We also know that pain is frightening. You may be afraid to move for fear that you're going to injure yourself further. You may worry that you're never going to function normally again. And you may be shaken when your doctor starts suggesting tests with high-tech, hard-to-pronounce names. This book aims to put you in charge of your pain and to remove the intimidation factor from common medical procedures.

About This Book

In our practice, we use a *whole-person, multidisciplinary approach.* When treating the whole person, we look at all the factors that contribute to back and neck pain. With a multidisciplinary approach, we often combine treatments from different disciplines – for instance, medical approaches, exercise, chiropractic, acupuncture, and bodywork – to help our patients overcome their back and neck pain problems. We believe that back and neck pain are completely manageable. We also believe that most people with back and neck pain don't need surgery.

Throughout this book, we look at both the physical and emotional causes, and ramifications, of back and neck pain. We show you ways to manage and relieve your pain, from aerobic exercises, nerve blocks, and medication to yoga and osteopathy. We also cover common treatments and diagnoses, and we look at the ways in which pain affects your life at home and at work.

Treating Your Back & Neck Pain For Dummies is organised in an easy-access manner. We start with the most basic information, such as an overview of back and neck and anatomy, and move through to more specific topics, including conventional and complementary treatments and rehabilitation.

This book's full of tips and anecdotes from our practice, many derived from our patients who've overcome the challenges of back and neck pain. You can find detailed explanations of common conditions, tests, and treatments – all described in plain English. (And if we ever do lapse into medical jargon, our editors make sure that we explain exactly what we mean in lay terms.)

Finally, this book's a tool that empowers you to get the best possible treatment – and results. We give you lists of questions to ask your practitioners, and we prepare you thoroughly for interaction with both the conventional and complementary medical communities. Say goodbye to the days of nodding your head as your doctor talks, only to wonder after the appointment what he or she meant. After all, when you're talking about your body, you deserve to be in control.

Foolish Assumptions

When we wrote this book, we made a few assumptions about you, the reader:

- ✔ You or someone you care about suffers from occasional, chronic, or recurring back or neck pain.
- ✔ You want to educate yourself about back and neck pain conditions and common treatments.
- ✔ You're frequently frustrated by the information – or lack of it – that you receive from the medical community.
- ✔ You want to take charge of your own treatment, and you want to make intelligent decisions about any tests or operations your practitioners suggest.
- ✔ You're interested in exploring some of the emotional aspects of living with back and neck pain.
- ✔ You want to feel better.
- ✔ You like chocolate ice cream. (You don't actually have to like chocolate ice cream, but we try to add a little humour here and there.)

What You're Not to Read

You don't have to read this book from cover to cover. Feel free to pick and choose and read what interests or applies to you and your situation. The book is *modular*, so you can start in the middle of Chapter 13 and then go to the beginning of Chapter 1 without losing any important information, and no matter how much you skip around, the book still makes sense. We've loaded the book with cross-references to other chapters, so you know precisely where to go for more info or further explanation of a term or treatment.

Of course, if you want to start at the beginning and read through to the end, go right ahead. The book does have a logical progression, so you can read from front to back if you prefer. Just remember that even though back and neck pain can be scary, we didn't write this book like an Agatha Christie thriller where you have to read every page. Use what you need, but skip the rest.

How This Book Is Organised

Remember in school when you had to provide your teachers with an outline of a chapter or a report? This book is organised in much the same way. We start out by dividing the text into parts, with each part covering a general area of back and neck pain and treatment. The parts are divided further into chapters. Each chapter deals with a specific issue that pertains to the entire part. Chapters are broken down by headings that separate the main ideas we cover, and sometimes we even use subheads. Our teachers would be so proud!

Part 1: Getting Back to Back and Neck Basics

This important part explains that back and neck pain are really common problems, and so you don't need to be embarrassed by your back or neck pain – millions of people face the same challenges. We spend a bit of time looking at spine anatomy and the causes of back and neck pain. This part ends with a chapter that suggests when you need to see a professional and what kind of practitioner can best help you.

Part 11: Conventional Treatment Options

We hate to hit you over the head with the obvious, but this part looks at conventional treatment options. When you first have a flare up of your pain, you may want to try some home remedies, so we talk about which of these may work in your situation. We also show you when to consider abandoning the home remedies for a visit to your GP.

Our goal is to help you make the best decision about your treatment. Doctors have several options for treating back and neck pain, and so we explain common tests and medical treatments for back and neck pain. We also devote a chapter to the surgical options. By the end of this part, you have all the tools you need to make intelligent decisions about your course of treatment.

Part III: Complementary Approaches: Are They for You?

If you have a mother or a financial advisor, you know that putting all your eggs in one basket is almost never a good idea. So in this part, we explore treatment options that you can use in conjunction with standard medical treatments, including the following (to name a few):

- Acupuncture
- Biofeedback
- Bodywork
- Massage
- Yoga

We spend some time discussing the mind–body connection and how you can use it to help manage your pain. No book on back and neck pain is complete without a chapter on osteopathy and chiropractic, and we're nothing if not thorough. We're also responsible, and so we show you how to recognise the charlatans out there who offer quick cures that only worsen your pain.

Part IV: Rehabilitation

This part gets into the hands-on stuff. We show you the exercises and treatments your doctor may recommend, and we walk through each of them with you. This part's also full of tips and tricks that you can do on your own to manage your pain and speed up recovery. We help you design an exercise programme tailored to your condition. Finally, we offer you a chapter on products that can make you and your back and neck more comfortable.

Part V: Resuming Normal Activity and Preventing Future Injury

Bet you can't guess what this part covers. Seriously though, as you are painfully aware, a bad back or neck can affect your overall quality of life. After you get the pain and the condition under control, returning to normal activities can be daunting. And after a siege of back or neck pain, you certainly want to prevent any future injuries. By following the tips in these chapters, you can safely return to work and engage in extra-curricular activities – all without fear of re-injury.

Part VI: The Part of Tens

All books in the *For Dummies* series contain a Part of Tens. These chapters offer titbits of information in easy bites. We cover ten (or so – *For Dummies* books aren't pedantic) of the following:

- ✔ Common questions about back and neck pain
- ✔ Steps to a healthy back and neck
- ✔ Reasons to see a doctor for back and neck pain
- ✔ Tips for working successfully with your practitioner

If nothing else, you're not going to run out of conversation topics at your next party.

Part VII: Appendixes

We end the book with two appendixes. The first is a glossary that gives you an at-a-glance definition of common terms in the world of back and neck pain treatments. The second is a list of resources and organisations that you can contact for further information and support.

Icons Used in This Book

As you thumb through this book, notice that we set off certain paragraphs with little icons. We use these icons to draw your attention to information that's especially important or that you may find particularly interesting. We use the following icons.

We occasionally add some information that's pretty technical in nature. If you really want to delve into the topic, you can enjoy the information we present here. Otherwise, feel free to skip these paragraphs.

You're not alone if your back or neck pain causes you anxiety. Paragraphs marked with this icon offer you healing or stress-relieving ideas.

This icon indicates things that we simply don't want you to forget.

This icon alerts you to those instances when you need to see your doctor.

We give our patients all kinds of tips for dealing with and managing their pain and their interaction with the medical community. We're happy to share these tips with you in the paragraphs marked with this icon.

This icon's not a picture of a bomb for nothing. These paragraphs warn you of things you mustn't do and symptoms you mustn't ignore. Think of these pieces of information as giant stop signs on the back and neck pain motorway.

Where to Go from Here

You've already made a commitment to helping yourself by getting this book. Just as you need to choose the best treatment options and remedies for you, you can now choose where to start reading. Take a look at the table of contents. When you find a topic that interests you, start reading your way to pain-free living.

Part I
Getting Back to Back and Neck Basics

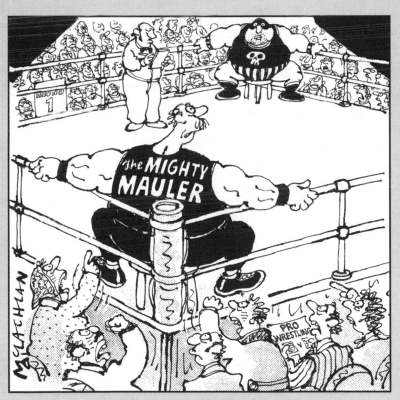

"Good Lord, Fiona, that's
my physiotherapist!"

In this part . . .

You are not suffering alone. Back and neck pain can be embarrassing and make you feel isolated from friends, coworkers – even your family. In this part, you discover just how common back and neck pain are – actually, almost everyone suffers from at least one bout of back or neck pain during his or her life. We also give you an overview of spinal anatomy, which is essential to understanding your pain, and we go on to discuss the things that can cause back and neck pain.

Chapter 1

Ouch! The Problem of Back and Neck Pain

· ·

In This Chapter

▶ Digging into the who, what, when, where, and why of back and neck pain

▶ Getting successful treatment

▶ Combining conventional and non-conventional treatments

· ·

*U*nless you find the topic of back and neck pain exciting, we imagine that you or someone you care about is experiencing back or neck pain. Finding appropriate treatment that actually works can be frustrating to say the least. And everybody seems to have an opinion about what you should do: Your mother-in-law swears by her chiropractor, your son thinks you should try yoga, your boss touts physiotherapy, and your best friend raves about the results of his surgery.

In addition to getting more advice than you want, you may notice that people treat you differently than people with other conditions. For example, how many times have you heard or said this sort of thing:

✔ You shouldn't lift those boxes without bending your knees: You'll hurt your back.

✔ You can't play golf – that twisting motion is bad for your back pain. You'll provoke an attack for certain.

✔ You have a bad neck or back! Don't even think about trying to sit in a cinema for two hours. In fact, you rest and we'll go out.

Even though back and neck pain is an incredibly common condition, the preceding examples illustrate just how much confusion surrounds the problem for both patients and health care professionals. If you've spent any time searching for a remedy to your back or neck pain, you're probably familiar with the bewildering number of opinions and treatment options out there. Two things cause this state of confusion:

- In most cases, the initial cause of the pain remains unknown.
- Health care providers disagree considerably over specific diagnoses and appropriate treatment plans.

These two problems mean you're likely to get a wide variety of diagnoses and treatment recommendations as you search for answers to your back or neck pain. In fact, the more you search, the more bewildered you may feel.

With all this conflicting information, you may not be sure which route to follow. Chapter 1 to the rescue! We start by giving you a solid definition of back and neck pain and go on to discuss treating the pain. Read on to get a grip on how back or neck pain applies to you.

Defining Back and Neck Pain

You may find the question 'What's back and neck pain?' odd. Your answer's probably along the lines of 'Pain in the back or neck of course!' However, as you may have experienced already, a general back or neck pain problem or a spinal condition can include many different symptoms.

We use the terms 'back and neck pain' and 'spinal condition' somewhat interchangeably. Sometimes, however, the terms mean different things. Back and neck pain are general terms and can be caused by a number of different reasons. Also, they're not limited to the back or neck but may be in the arms and legs as well. A spinal condition does not always cause back or neck pain.

If you have back or neck pain or a spinal condition, you may experience a variety of symptoms, including:

- Pain with a throbbing, aching, shooting, stabbing, dull, or sharp quality.
- Pain down one or both legs, with very little pain in the lower back.
- Numbness or weakness in the legs.
- Pain in the lower back and legs that occurs only in certain positions.
- Sleep problems, decreased energy, depression, and anxiety.
- Pain that seems to move to different parts of the body, including the back or neck.
- Pain brought on or worsened by stress and emotional issues.

The preceding examples represent just a few of the many ways in which back and neck pain problems present themselves. To get good treatment and ensure that treatment doesn't actually make your problem worse, you need a good understanding of the different types of back and neck pain problems (see Chapter 3 for details). This knowledge helps you gain control over your particular problem.

Who experiences back and neck pain?

Back and neck pain are very common conditions. Many doctors and researchers consider back and neck pain to be a normal part of life, similar to having an occasional cold or sore throat. As a person with back or neck pain, you're not alone. In the UK:

- Back pain affects more than 80 per cent of the population at some time during their lifetime.
- Back pain is second only to the common cold as a reason for visits to the doctor and second only to childbirth as a reason for hospitalisation.
- Back problems are reported by approximately 50 per cent of the working population every year.
- Back and neck pain costs approximately 10 billion pounds a year in the UK.
- Back pain is often accompanied by neck pain: About 60 per cent of people with back pain also have neck problems.

What causes back and neck pain?

Back and neck pain have a great many known medical causes (see Chapter 3 for details). If you venture outside the realm of conventional Western medicine, the list of possible reasons for spinal pain becomes even longer. For the purposes of the discussion in this section, we present only a few examples of the more common causes of back and neck pain.

One point – that most practitioners often ignore – is absolutely critical: When you're investigating the various possible reasons for your pain, remember that all pain has both physical *and* emotional components. If you ignore the physical or the emotional influences, you're less likely to find a remedy. We discuss the components of pain in Chapter 3.

Probably the most important thing to keep in mind regarding the causes of back and neck pain is that doctors don't determine an exact reason for the majority of spinal pain problems. Even so, don't be discouraged: Most back and neck pain problems resolve completely, even when the exact cause is unknown.

One of the most common causes of back and neck pain includes problems with the muscles and ligaments. Similar to other tissues in your body, the muscles and ligaments of your back or neck can be injured, irritated, or weakened, which then causes pain.

Another cause of back and neck pain, which often appears in conjunction with pain down one or both legs, is a disc problem. Two common disc problems are *disc bulge* and *disc herniation*. *Discs* are 'cushions' lying between each of the *vertebrae* (the bones of your back) (see Chapter 2). Problems occur when part of the disc *bulges* (pushes out) or *herniates* (breaks through) out of its usual space and presses, or comes close to nerves that go down your legs. This pressing and irritation of the nerve is why some back problems cause pain down your legs. Pain can result even if the disc isn't actually pressing on the nerve but only comes in close proximity. Chemicals released by the disc make the nerve sensitive and can cause pain.

We'd be remiss if we didn't mention that 'disc bulge' and 'disc herniation' are no longer the current medical terms for describing disc problems. In the ever-changing area of medical terminology, the new labels are disc protrusion and disc extrusion. A *disc protrusion* is roughly equivalent to a bulge, and *disc extrusion* approximates the definition of a herniation. (You find some other, very slight technical differences between the old and new terms, but nothing that would ever come up in ordinary conversation.) Even though the terms protrusion and extrusion are more technically correct, we generally use the terms bulge and herniation in this book. Also, the labels of bulging and herniation are still the most commonly used terms by health professionals, both in practice and in books on back and neck pain.

Another common factor in the continuation back and neck pain (and one which we believe doctors often miss) is stress. In this case, back and neck pain starts, is maintained, or is worsened by emotionally stressful experiences. Stress (conscious or unconscious) can cause your muscles to tighten, which then causes pain. Stress can also amplify the amount of pain coming from some other back or neck problem, such as a herniated disc. Consequently, paying attention to both the emotional and physical aspects of back pain is very important.

Treating Back and Neck Pain

As you try to manage your pain problem and investigate various treatment approaches, help yourself by being assured and hopeful that you *can* remedy your problem. Back and neck pain do get better, and successful treatment is possible. You can find the best treatment for your problem when you have some understanding of who treats back and neck pain, how they treat it, and why using a multidisciplinary approach is important.

My back or neck pain can get better, can't it?

Although back and neck problems are very common, the good news is that generally they resolve on their own. In fact, the usual outcome of spinal pain symptoms is very favourable, often with or without treatment.

Determining which treatments are and aren't successful is often challenging because of the natural tendency of spinal pain to improve – the pain often goes away on its own, regardless of whether you receive treatment. However, even with the human body's natural pattern towards improvement, many people with back or neck pain experience pain that lingers, worsens, or seems to come and go. If you're reading this book, odds are that your back or neck pain problem falls into the category of not getting better on its own. Here are some of the more common pain situations:

- ✔ Flare ups of back or neck pain that seem to come and go over several years.

- ✔ Chronic back or neck pain problems that go on for more than three months.

- ✔ Back and neck pain for which the recommendation is surgery.

- ✔ Back or leg pain that continues even after spinal surgery (this type of pain is called *failed low-back surgery syndrome*).

The preceding types of pain don't resolve themselves quickly and can become increasingly frustrating for you and those close to you. Getting accurate information about your back or neck pain problem is your most important resource for getting better.

Often, the appropriate timing and integration of treatment options – conventional or non-conventional – is the key for you to overcome your pain problem successfully. For example, you may improve with physiotherapy treatments such as electrical stimulation, ice, and heat in combination with an exercise programme and acupuncture if you receive all these treatments in a specific overlapping timeframe.

The importance of treatment integration also involves surgery, which may or may not be effective depending on a number of factors. Spinal surgery is appropriate in certain cases. You can improve the chances of having a good outcome if you add treatments such as psychological preparation for surgery (undergoing relaxation training, gathering information about your surgery, and having a healthy attitude towards the operation) and post-operative rehabilitation (exercise, psychological techniques, and complementary medicine approaches) to your treatment programme. (See Chapter 8 for more on psychological preparation for surgery and Chapters 12 and 14 for more on post-operative rehabilitation.)

Who can treat my back or neck pain?

A variety of practitioners treat back and neck pain problems by using medical and non-medical approaches. Although many specialties are involved in the evaluation and treatment of back and neck pain, the following specialties are common. This list is in alphabetical order and doesn't imply that you should proceed in this order when seeking treatment for your back or neck pain. Actually, we recommend starting your treatment with a general type of practitioner, such as your GP, physiotherapist, chiropractor, or osteopath, and then moving on to specialists as required, such as a rheumatologist, orthopaedic surgeon, or neurosurgeon. (We discuss the following specialties in greater detail in Chapter 4.)

- **Anaesthetics:** This area of medical practice focuses on decreasing or abolishing the patient's sensation of pain. Some anaesthetists have specialised training in treating pain problems and are often involved in running pain clinics. The treatment approach may include such things as medications, spinal injections, and general anaesthesia (inducing a state that allows for surgical intervention). For more about anaesthetic pain treatments, see Chapter 7.

- **Chiropractic:** This system of evaluation and treatment is based upon the belief that abnormal function of the nervous system causes disease. Chiropractors try to restore normal function by treating and manipulating different body parts, especially the spine. As well as manipulation, most chiropractors provide a variety of other treatments such as massage, nutritional counselling, and vitamin therapy. We describe chiropractic in detail in Chapter 11.

- **General practice:** Your GP is your family, or primary care, doctor and is usually the first professional you consult for a back or neck pain problem. Because many cases of back and neck pain get better without treatment or with minimal treatment, your GP is fully equipped to handle your problem initially. GPs have general training in all areas of medicine, but if you need a more specialised approach, he or she can refer you to an appropriate specialist.

- **Neurology:** This branch of medicine deals with the nervous system. Neurologists often use non-surgical treatment approaches to diagnose and treat back pain. Chapter 4 has more about neurology.

- **Neurosurgery:** This medical specialty focuses on the surgical treatment of nervous system problems. A neurosurgeon generally uses a surgical treatment approach and may be involved in such things as removing tumours from the brain and repairing damaged nerves after a severe injury. Neurosurgeons who specialise in spine problems use a surgical treatment approach (see Chapter 9 for more information about spine surgery).

✔ **Orthopaedic surgery:** This area of medicine focuses on the surgical treatment of skeletal problems. For example, general orthopaedic surgeons perform hip and knee replacement surgery, repair severely fractured bones, and undertake other types of joint surgery. Some orthopaedic surgeons specialise in the treatment and surgery of spinal problems and may remove discs or fuse spinal joints together.

✔ **Osteopathy:** This system is very similar to chiropractic but also emphasises *body mechanics* (for example, your posture while being still or moving – see Chapter 14) and manipulative techniques (such as moving or adjusting your joints – see Chapter 11).

✔ **Pain psychology:** This discipline is a specialised branch of clinical psychology that uses psychological methods to diagnose and treat pain problems. Examples include helping you identify thoughts or emotions that make your back pain worse, teaching you relaxation exercises, and helping you change your attitude towards the pain. (For more details about pain psychology treatment, check out Chapter 13.)

✔ **Cognitive Behavioural Therapy:** CBT is a collection of techniques, which address the sometimes disabling effects of back and neck pain. The *cognitive* aspect uses clinical psychology to address the thoughts or emotions that reduce your ability to cope with and manage your pain most effectively. These thoughts and feelings can make your back pain worse and can increase the disability you experience. The *behavioural* aspect looks at the way people react to pain and promotes the activities that are most positive, such as keeping active, and returning to work. It does not encourage behaviour that's not helpful long-term such as using a stick, limping, and resting for long periods. CBT programmes help you change your attitude towards the pain.

✔ **Rheumatology:** This branch of medicine deals with disorders of the musculo-skeletal system, particularly inflammatory diseases such as rheumatoid arthritis. Many consultant rheumatologists are also involved with back and neck pain. Chapter 4 has more about rheumatology.

✔ **Physiotherapy:** This uses hands-on treatments such as manual therapy or manipulation, electrical treatments, education, and specialised exercise to treat pain and disability. Physiotherapists also use aspects of behavioural therapy to encourage a return to normality or as close to normal as you can get.

How is my back or neck pain treated?

Your doctor or specialist may recommend you try a variety of other treatments, such as the following:

- **Braces, corsets, and collars:** These items may be useful but in the majority of cases should only be used short-term (a week or two). They restrict motion, provide support, and may decrease your back and neck pain. You can buy general back supports and collars without a prescription at many pharmacies or on the Internet. Your GP or specialist physician can also prescribe other types of brace. Your doctor or physiotherapist should always guide your use of a back brace or collar (for more info, see Chapters 8).

- **Exercise:** Exercise is probably one of the most important treatments for back pain. Your doctor may recommend different types of exercise programmes for your back or neck pain, including lumbar stabilisation and cardiovascular conditioning. We discuss these techniques more fully in Chapter 15.

- **Medication:** Doctors use a variety of drugs to treat back pain including *analgesics* (painkillers), anti-inflammatories, and muscle relaxants. The doctor most involved in treating your back or neck pain problem usually prescribes these medications, but sometimes your specialist (such as an orthopaedic surgeon) asks your GP to manage your medications because he or she is more familiar with your medical history.

- **Pain management:** This treatment combines a variety of approaches – including psychological avenues such as CBT, medicines, exercise, and working with family members – to address your pain problem. The doctor most involved in your back or neck pain treatment usually recommends the treatment combinations, but you may decide to add treatments yourself.

- **Physiotherapy:** Your doctor may prescribe physiotherapy from a physiotherapist for your back or neck pain problem. Examples of treatment include special exercises, manual therapy or manipulation, deep-tissue massage, heat and cold treatments, hydrotherapy, and treatments that use electrical stimulation. See Chapter 4 for more about physiotherapy.

- **Spinal epidural steroid and nerve blocks:** These treatments involve injecting drugs – usually steroids or anaesthetics – into a particular area of the spinal canal to help your back or neck pain and nerve irritation. (See Chapter 7 for more about this treatment.)

- **Stress management and posture:** Stress management such as relaxation training, yoga, and thought analysis can help with back and neck pain problems (see Chapters 11 and 12 for more info). Addressing your posture in your work or home environment can also be an important part of your treatment (see Chapter 14).

✔ **Trigger point therapy:** This treatment involves massaging or injecting a small amount of anaesthetic painkiller or other medicine such as local steroids into *trigger points*, the areas of a muscle that seem to trigger pain in a given region of the body. It is easily self-administered and can be extremely useful.

Diagnostic and treatment approaches not normally associated with mainstream medicine are termed *non-conventional*, *alternative*, or *complementary* medicine approaches. We believe complementary treatment approaches definitely have a place in the treatment of back and neck pain problems. In this book we use the term 'complementary' to describe these approaches because this term best describes how we believe you should incorporate them into a pain treatment programme: These treatments should always be a *complement* rather than an *alternative* to medical management. Incorporating mainstream medical management and complementary approaches is the only safe way to combine these different treatment philosophies. We discuss the specifics of safely pursuing complementary medicine treatments in Chapter 10. Here are some examples of the more common complementary treatments:

✔ **Acupuncture:** In this ancient Chinese medicine approach, the acupuncturist uses small needles to pierce the skin at specific body locations (*acupoints*) to cause healing and other benefits, such as pain relief (for more details on acupuncture, see Chapter 10).

✔ **Alexander Technique:** Qualified Alexander Technique specialists analyse your body positions and the way you move. Through instruction and practise, you can correct movement patterns, which relieves unnecessary stress and strain on your body.

✔ **Aromatherapy:** This treatment involves the use of essential oils from plants for healing and relaxation. The oils are believed to have pain-relieving properties.

✔ **Bodywork:** Therapies such as massage, deep-tissue manipulation, movement awareness, and energy balancing can improve the body's structure and function and reduce pain.

✔ **Chiropractic:** This treatment aims to influence the body's nervous system and ability to heal through adjustments of the spine, muscles, and joints and other treatment approaches (for more info, check out Chapter 11).

✔ **Mind–body approaches:** A number of different approaches can promote the body's own ability to heal itself and increase the mind's power over the body. We talk about a number of these treatments in Chapter 13.

✔ **Osteopathy:** Osteopathic approaches and treatments are very similar to those of chiropractic.

- **Reflexology, or reflex zone therapy:** This therapy is a specialised foot massage based on a system of energy pathways. Many people report that reflexology helps their back and neck pain.

- **T'ai chi:** This Chinese system of physical movement is designed to harmonise the individual with the forces of nature. People with spinal pain often find it useful to encourage movement and flexibility in the body. Head to Chapter 10 to find out more about t'ai chi.

- **Yoga:** This system of health uses physical postures, breathing exercises, and meditation to relieve suffering and enhance overall wellbeing. We discuss yoga approaches for back pain in Chapter 12.

How do I choose a multidisciplinary approach?

A *multidisciplinary approach* is the combining of a variety of treatment approaches to address a spinal pain problem. Research shows that back and neck pain problems, especially those that aren't improving, respond best to a combination of different approaches delivered in a co-ordinated fashion. If your pain isn't responding to a single approach such as an exercise programme or medication, you may want to consider a multidisciplinary approach.

You can get multidisciplinary treatment for your pain in a number of ways. For instance, you can participate in a structured *pain management programme* in which the treatment components (such as exercise, relaxation, medicines, cognitive therapy, and so on) are delivered in a group format to a number of people with ongoing pain. A medical director generally oversees and co-ordinates the treatment in these programmes, which aren't very common and are usually based within a hospital setting.

Other multidisciplinary treatment approaches are less formal and less structured than pain programmes. The informal multidisciplinary approach takes many forms, and the types of treatment that are combined differ from person to person. Your doctor may help you construct an individually tailored multidisciplinary programme. In this situation, your doctor works with you to determine the best treatments and assists you in co-ordinating these treatments.

 Unfortunately, many doctors don't think in terms of a multidisciplinary approach and you may have to design and co-ordinate your own programme. You can still have a good outcome – you just have to work a little harder. The information in this book gives you an idea of the various treatments available as well as those that may address your particular back or neck pain problem.

A multidisciplinary approach for back or neck pain may include the following:

✔ **Body mechanics and ergonomics:** This treatment encourages you to use good posture and makes sure your work area is safe for your back and neck (see Chapter 13 for more on this subject).

✔ **Complementary approaches:** Complementary medicinal approaches often form part of a treatment programme for back and neck pain. They may include, among other things, yoga and acupuncture.

✔ **Medical management:** Your doctor, osteopath, or chiropractor responsible for prescribing the treatment components may oversee a multidisciplinary treatment programme. Alternatively, you may put together your own multidisciplinary programme. If a doctor oversees your treatment, he or she may be responsible for prescribing any medications, manual medical techniques, invasive procedures, and physiotherapy exercises that you need.

✔ **Physiotherapy:** Many multidisciplinary treatment approaches include an aggressive rehabilitation programme focusing on muscular *reconditioning* (strengthening) especially around your lower back area. A physiotherapist may also use physiotherapy *modalities*; techniques to relieve pain such as hot and cold packs, ultrasound, and massage. Check out Chapter 4 for more about physiotherapy.

✔ **Stress and pain management:** A pain psychologist can show you home techniques for relaxation and help you gain insights into the role that stress plays in your back pain (see Chapters 3 and 9 for more on this subject).

Although your back or neck pain may improve when working with a single practitioner, sometimes an individual specialist can't adequately treat a difficult pain problem and its associated complications. In a multidisciplinary treatment, you complete all appropriate treatments simultaneously in a co-ordinated fashion, which offers better results than going through one treatment at a time.

Chapter 2

Introducing the Parts of Your Spine

. . . .

In This Chapter

▶ Recognising your spine's strong structure

▶ Increasing your awareness of your spine

▶ Understanding how the parts of your spine work together

. . . .

*Y*ou know where your spine is, but you may have no idea what it actually looks like. This chapter acquaints you with your spine and helps you understand the various terms your doctor, or medically trained practitioner, may use when discussing your back pain.

This chapter prepares you to 'talk the talk' with your practitioner when it comes to your spine. Don't panic if your doctor tells you that you have lumbar sacral sprain-strain injury – this complex phrase simply means you have a sore muscle or joint in your lower back, and with the proper treatment (such as time to heal and appropriate exercise) you can get back to normal life.

Being familiar with the language of spinal anatomy helps you:

✔ Ask pertinent questions

✔ Get meaningful answers

✔ Obtain the correct treatment

As you explore the parts of your spine, don't worry that you have every disease you've ever read about. Having a little knowledge can make things worse: We've had patients study their spines, only to worry that each area they studied was weak or malfunctioning.

As you read this chapter, remember five important things:

- **Extensive sets of muscles and ligaments support your spine, creating a very strong yet mobile structure:** Your spine's very flexible, allowing you to bend forward, backwards, and sideways, while supporting your head (which weighs 6–8 kilograms) and your torso (45–62 kilograms). Your lower spine has a *lifting capacity* (the weight up to which you can lift) of up to 150 kilograms per 6.5 square centimetres (300 pounds per square inch). For a pile of bones strung together with ligaments and muscles, that's truly an amazing feat.

- **Doctors identify no specific structural problem in the majority of people with back or neck pain:** The structure of your spine is usually in good shape and your pain is most likely not due to anything life-threatening or that requires surgery. Your pain will respond to appropriate treatment and exercise.

- **Surgery is very rarely necessary in order to become pain free:** In fact, in the UK, only a tiny percentage of patients with back or neck pain come to surgery.

- **Effective treatment is possible without a specific diagnosis:** Common principles such as keeping as active as possible and remaining positive help you to focus on getting better rather than searching for a diagnosis.

- **Structural abnormalities such as a herniated disc often have nothing to do with your pain:** For example, a large percentage of adults with no back pain have bulging or herniated discs, meaning that a condition like a herniated disc is not necessarily causing your pain (see Chapter 3).

Feeling Fine with Help from Your Spine

Have you ever wondered why you have a spine and what it does? Probably not, but the subject is fascinating. Really! Your spine serves several purposes:

- **Your spine supports your upper body:** Your spine supports the weight of your head and upper body, allowing you to do things like read this book.

- **Your spine provides flexibility:** Your spine supports your upper body so you can bend forwards, backwards, and sideways. Life would be a bit more challenging if your spine was a straight rigid pole from your hips to your head.

✔ **Your spine houses and protects your spinal cord and nerves:** Your spine encloses your spinal cord, which is a relay station of nerves going to and from your brain to all parts of your body. Your spine also acts as a protective covering so that these nerves aren't damaged as you move around.

✔ **Your spine serves as an attachment for muscles and ligaments:** Your spine's one of your skeleton's basic building blocks. Without your spine to provide an attachment for many of your torso's muscles and ligaments, your upper body would fall into a shapeless pile of tissue.

✔ **Your spine serves as a platform for your head:** If you didn't have a spine, where would you put your head?

Don't take the engineering marvel that's your spine for granted. Your spine continues to provide you with all the features just mentioned when you're in pain. The following section offers you a chance to become more familiar with the amazing intricacies of your spine.

Touring Your Splendid Spine

The rest of this chapter discusses the various parts of your spine. You can divide your spinal structures into the following:

✔ The spinal column

✔ The vertebrae

✔ The discs (also called intervertebral discs)

✔ The facet joints

✔ The ligaments

✔ The spinal canal (which is nowhere near the Panama Canal)

✔ The sacrum and coccyx

✔ The sacroiliac joints (SI joints)

✔ The nerves

✔ The muscles

✔ The vertebral arteries (blood vessels)

The spinal column

Your back divides into three natural curves that form an S-shape (see Figure 2-1): The cervical curve, containing your neck bones; the thoracic curve, containing the bones of your middle back; and the lumbosacral curve, containing the bones of your lower back.

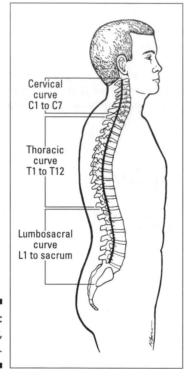

Figure 2-1:
Your curvy,
bony spine.

When all your spine's curves are in balance (refer to Figure 2-1), your ear, shoulder, and hip align to make a straight line, even though your back curves between these points. *Good posture* means keeping your back curves in balance (see Chapter 14 for more about posture).

The vertebrae: the bones of your back

The bones of your spine are called *vertebrae* (each individual bone is called a *vertebra*). The vertebrae are some of the most important parts of your spine. You have a total of 24 vertebrae in your back:

✔ The cervical part of your spine contains seven vertebrae, which support the weight of your head and protect the nerves that come from your brain to the rest of your body. In technical terms, medical people refer to these vertebrae as C1–C7, with C1 being the vertebra just under your head. Your cervical vertebrae literally keep your head on your shoulders.

✔ The thoracic part of your spine contains 12 vertebrae, making up your mid-back. Those in the know refer to these bones as T1–T12.

✔ The lumbosacral spine contains the five vertebrae in your lower back and sacrum. No surprises here – the lumbar vertebrae go from L1 to L5. The lumbosacral curve is your spine's workhorse, moving more than the rest of your spine (except your neck) and carrying the majority of the weight of your body.

A vertebra has three parts: the vertebral body, the transverse process, and the spinous process.

Figure 2-2 shows two vertebrae with a disc in between (see the next section for more about discs). The *vertebral body* is the large front part of the vertebra that is cushioned by the discs. The *spinous process* is the part of the vertebrae that you can feel as the bony bumps on your back. The *transverse process* provides an area of attachment for the muscles that control your spine's movement. Also notice the opening through which the spinal cord passes, termed the *spinal canal*.

The discs

Lying in between each of the vertebral bodies, the *discs* are your spine's cushioning pads or 'shock absorbers.' Figure 2-2 shows two vertebrae with a disc in between. Together, two vertebrae and a disc are known as a *functional unit*. Figure 2-3 shows a cut-away view of a functional unit.

As we show in Figure 2-4, two parts make up the disc:

✔ **Nucleus pulposus:** This spongy centre provides lubrication and shock absorption for your spinal column, allowing some flexibility in between each vertebra while also providing shock absorption to the structures of your spine (including the nerves). The nucleus pulposus is mostly made up of water, so it's very flexible.

✔ **Annulus fibrosis:** This outer layer attaches to and holds together the vertebrae. The annulus fibrosis is very tough and has a criss-cross design.

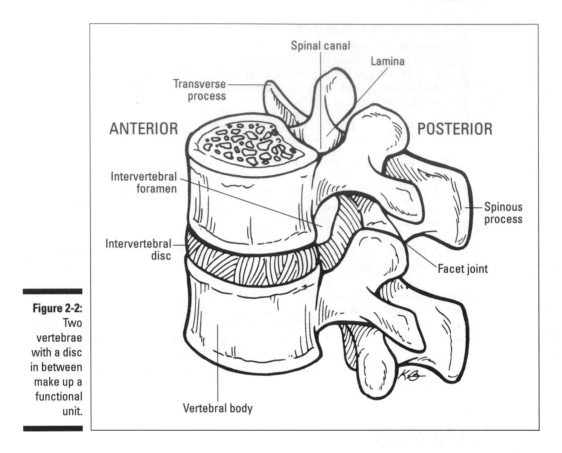

Figure 2-2:
Two vertebrae with a disc in between make up a functional unit.

The disc's design allows the bony vertebrae to move back and forth, giving your spine great flexibility, like the links of one of those jointed toy snakes.

The facet joints

If you refer to Figure 2-2, you see a *facet joint* – a gliding joint – between each vertebra. Facet joints keep the vertebrae in alignment as your spine moves. Surrounding and enclosing the facet joints are joint capsules consisting of a smooth lining called *synovium*. The synovium produces synovial fluid, which helps lubricate the facet joint ensuring smooth movement. The synovial fluid also provides nourishment to the ends of the bones in the facet joint.

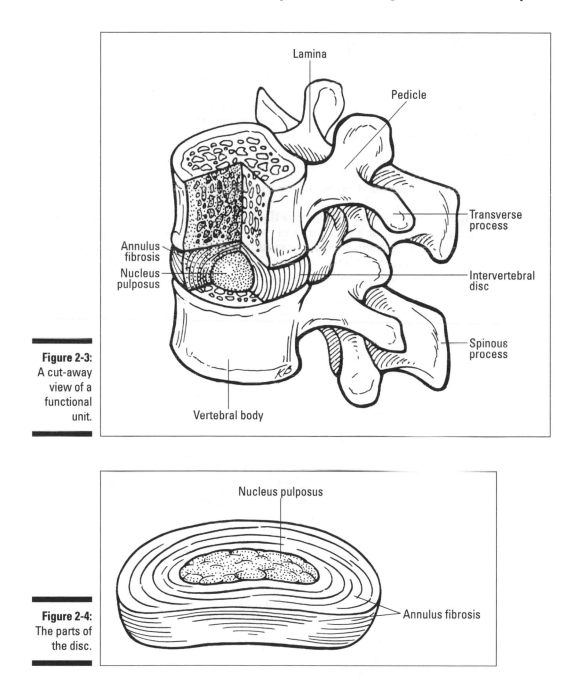

Figure 2-3:
A cut-away
view of a
functional
unit.

Figure 2-4:
The parts of
the disc.

The ligaments

As shown in Figure 2-5, your spine has more ligaments than anyone cares to know about – except maybe a back doctor. *Ligaments* are strong bands of fibrous tissue that knit your bones together and also contain pain fibres. At this point, we discuss just two of the ligaments that may be implicated in back and neck pain problems:

- The anterior (towards the front) longitudinal ligament
- The posterior (towards the rear) longitudinal ligament

These ligaments connect together the functional units (refer to 'The discs' section earlier in this chapter) and go up and down the entire length of your spine. They also help control the motion of your spine while providing flexibility. If you think of all the ligaments in your spine as sailors, these two are the captain and first mate.

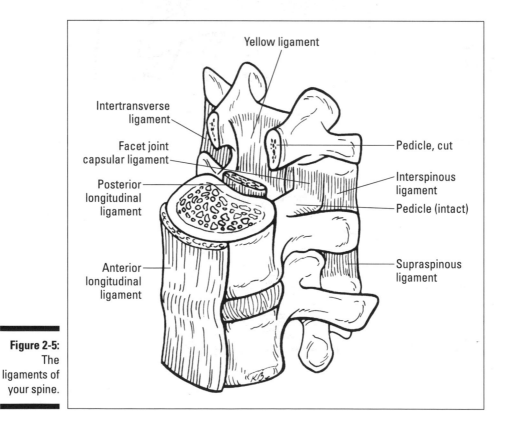

Figure 2-5:
The
ligaments of
your spine.

The spinal canal

Because your vertebrae are aligned on top of one another, they form an opening called the spinal canal (refer to Figure 2-2). The spinal cord passes through the canal and is protected by the bony vertebrae.

The sacrum and the coccyx

Below the five lumbar vertebrae, five more vertebrae are joined (fused) together. These five vertebrae make up the *sacrum* (see Figure 2-6), which forms the back part of your pelvis and the lowest part of your lumbosacral curve. Most people have five lumbar vertebrae and five fused sacral vertebrae. In a few people, the top sacral vertebra does not fuse with the other four sacral bones, resulting in six lumbar vertebrae and four fused sacral vertebrae. If you're one of these rare people, don't worry: This condition is rarely the cause of any back problems.

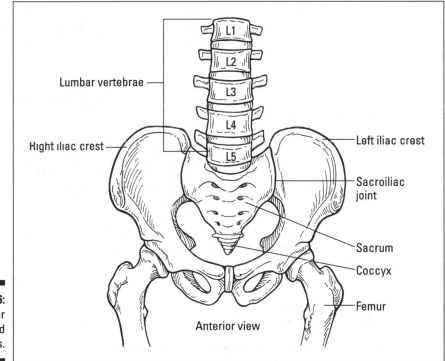

Figure 2-6:
The lumbar spine and pelvis.

The *coccyx* – the very bottom structure of the bony part of your spine – consists of three to five small vertebrae attached to the bottom of the sacrum. The coccyx may be more familiar to you as your *tailbone*. Injury to this very sensitive area can result in a painful condition called *coccydynia*, which we discuss in Chapter 3.

The sacroiliac joints

The *sacroiliac joints* are the joints that attach the sacrum to the *iliac bones* – your hip bones – of the pelvis (refer to Figure 2-6). The hip bones are attached to the sacrum by a number of ligaments on either side. To feel your iliac bones, just place your hands on your hips.

The spinal nerves

The *spinal cord* is made up of nerves that extend from the brain into the spinal canal and then out to the various parts of the body. The spinal canal is formed by the large part of the vertebrae as well as other structures. *Cerebral spinal fluid* (CSF) – the same fluid you find in the centre of the brain – partly fills the tube-like spinal canal. CSF helps protect the spinal cord within the spinal canal.

Figure 2-7 shows the *nerve roots*, where nerves leave your spine at various places. The nerves leave the spinal cord at different points and go out to the various parts of the body.

Figure 2-8 shows a close-up view of the spinal cord, nerve roots, and the spinal nerve branches. A nerve pain problem can be caused by a *disc bulge* or herniation. In this condition, part of the disc bulges or herniates out of its usual space and presses on one or more nerves. If herniation occurs in the neck area, you often feel pain down your arms and in your fingers. This pain is often described as sharp, shooting, electrical, or tingling. If a disc herniation occurs in the lower back, it may cause pain and/or tingling in the buttocks, legs, and feet. This condition is called sciatica. (Chapter 3 has more about disc bulge and sciatica.)

The muscles

The spine's functioning involves a great many muscles, including those in the back and abdominal areas. This section reviews only the most important muscles involved in spine function and back pain problems.

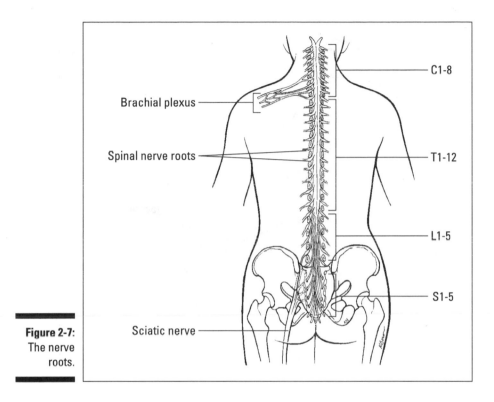

Brachial plexus —

Spinal nerve roots —

Sciatic nerve —

C1-8

T1-12

L1-5

S1-5

Figure 2-7:
The nerve
roots.

The *erector spinae* muscles (see Figure 2-9) are the muscles you feel on either side of your lower spine. When your doctor talks about muscle spasms in your back, these muscles are usually the culprits. Just under these long muscles are medium-length muscles that extend from one vertebra to the next. Underneath these are even shorter muscles that attach to the facet joints.

At the front of your body, the *psoas muscle* runs from the front and sides of your lower spine, goes across the hip joint, and attaches to the upper part of the *femur* (thigh bone).

The front of your body houses the all-important *abdominal muscles*. These muscles are critical to your spine's forward movement. They also provide support, which is why physiotherapists often instruct you to focus on strengthening your abdominal muscles as part of a back pain rehabilitation programme.

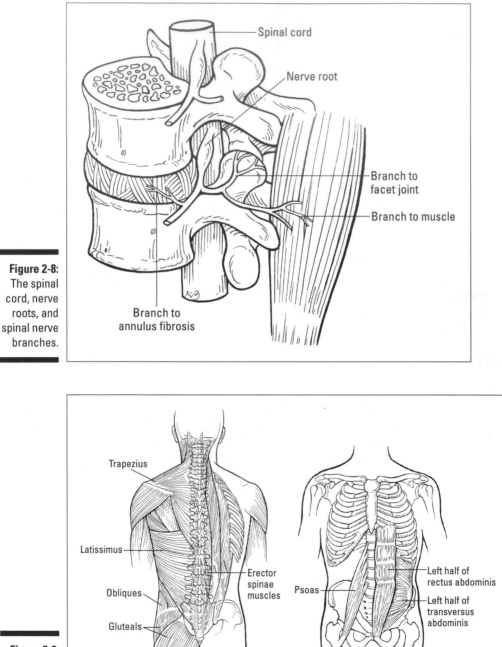

Figure 2-8: The spinal cord, nerve roots, and spinal nerve branches.

Spinal cord

Nerve root

Branch to facet joint

Branch to muscle

Branch to annulus fibrosis

Figure 2-9: The muscles.

Trapezius

Latissimus

Obliques

Gluteals

Erector spinae muscles

Psoas

Left half of rectus abdominis

Left half of transversus abdominis

The vertebral arteries

As shown in Figure 2-10, the vertebral arteries are the source of blood supply to your brain. Each artery naturally kinks before it enters your skull. Some movements, such as fully turning the head to left or right, temporarily block one of these arteries. This doesn't matter, as long as the other artery isn't restricted. If you have arterial disease, which is fairly common in older people, both of your vertebral arteries may be restricted – blockage in one artery can then cause problems, such as collapse. Treatment for some spinal pain may involve manipulation of the neck. This shouldn't be done if you have arterial disease because of the risk and possible fatal consequences of cutting off the blood supply to the brain. If you get dizzy when standing up or turning suddenly (a symptom of arterial disease), manipulation isn't for you.

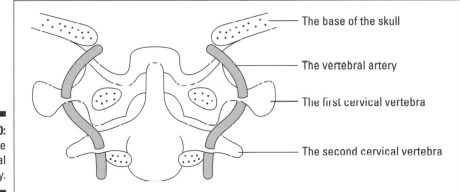

Figure 2-10: The vertebral artery.

The base of the skull

The vertebral artery

The first cervical vertebra

The second cervical vertebra

Chapter 3

Examining the Nature and Causes of Back and Neck Pain

In This Chapter

▶ Realising that back and neck pain features physical, mental, and emotional factors

▶ Understanding why you hurt

▶ Getting information on your diagnosis

▶ Exploring conditions that cause back and neck pain

Contrary to popular belief, all pain is real. Unfortunately, many people with back or neck pain are treated as if their pain is imaginary or exaggerated. We've seen patients who've had their pain dismissed so often by friends and family that they feel the need to 'prove' the pain to us. Some doctors also try to convince patients that because they can't find a physical cause for the pain, the pain can't be that bad. If this happens to you, get a second opinion from a practitioner who takes your pain seriously.

This problem arises because no medical tests are available to measure pain levels, so doctors can't test for pain in the same way they can test for a broken leg (with an X-ray) or an infection (with a blood test). To make matters more challenging, in people with back or neck pain, there's often little or no physical evidence to explain the pain. People with back or neck pain often go from one doctor to the next, searching for explanations, struggling through one unnecessary evaluation after another and never-ending treatments. We know of instances in which well-meaning but poorly informed health care professionals treated back or neck pain incorrectly and as a result harmed their patients.

Along with the general public, many doctors also misunderstand back and neck pain.

A valuable tool in discovering how to control your pain – and the crucial first step to recovery – is understanding why you hurt. In this chapter we look at one view of how pain works: The gate control theory.

Discovering the Gate Control Theory of Pain

Why do some people with serious injuries experience little pain, whereas others with relatively minor injuries suffer far more? Why do mind–body techniques such as hypnosis control pain? How do negative thoughts (being pessimistic) and emotions (being depressed) make your pain worse? And how can being optimistic and happy alleviate your pain? These difficult questions were answered by the *gate control theory of pain* developed in the early 1960s by two doctors, Ronald Melzack and Patrick Wall. The gate control theory explains that your thoughts, emotions, and physical factors (such as inactivity) can influence pain. As illustrated in Figure 3-1, nerve gates, or *pain gates*, in your spinal cord open and close depending on messages coming down from your brain (along the descending spinal nerves). If the pain gates are more open, the pain message flows freely and you experience more pain. If the gates are more closed, your pain is reduced or even stopped.

The gate control theory is complex, but the message it offers is simple and empowering: You can control your experience of pain. The gate control theory is also extremely important because it explains how all the different remedies for back and neck pain work, including both mental and physical techniques.

In the gate control theory of pain, the pain signal is transmitted through the *peripheral nervous system* (the nervous system outside of your brain and spinal cord) to the *central nervous system* (which includes the spinal cord and brain). In the spinal cord, the pain gates determine how much of the pain message gets through to the pain-sensation centre of the brain where you actually 'feel' the pain (in Figure 3-1 the pain signal starts in the foot). After the pain signal reaches your brain, it may be amplified or minimised depending on your thoughts, emotions, and physical factors, such as your overall health and conditioning. Figure 3-1 shows how the thought and emotional centres of your brain influence the pain gates and the pain-sensation centre.

The gate control theory

Imagine that you're crossing the road and you step on something that badly cuts your foot. Ouch! The pain is pretty bad. Now imagine that a car is coming towards you. The pain gate closes and you stop feeling the pain in your foot so you can quickly get out of the way. The pain only comes back when you're safely out of the road.

The pain gates are opened and the pain signal amplified (more pain overall) by such things as pessimistic thoughts, fear of the pain, hopelessness, depression, anxiety, and inactivity. The pain gates are closed and the pain signal minimised by such things as optimistic thoughts, distracting yourself from the pain, outside interests, taking control of your life, and physical conditioning.

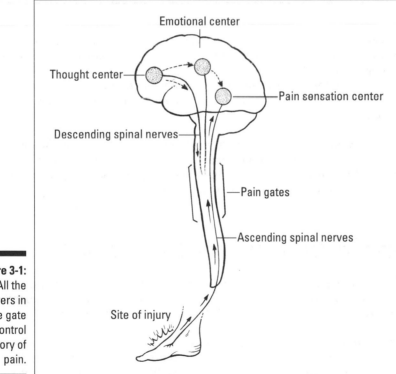

Figure 3-1:
All the players in the gate control theory of pain.

Open pain gates create a crisis

Dr Sinel (one of the authors of this book) had a patient at Cornell University Medical Center who came in complaining of headaches, which she described as severely painful and debilitating. The patient couldn't make it through the day without narcotic pain medicine. A thorough neurological examination and history proved to be entirely normal.

On further questioning, the patient revealed that her husband had recently been diagnosed with an inoperable brain tumour. She said that his initial symptoms were headaches, for which he had failed to seek medical advice for three months. A brain tumour was ultimately diagnosed, and the patient's husband died shortly afterwards.

This patient's extreme fear that she also had a brain tumour made her nervous system think that she might be in danger, the pain gates opened up, causing intense suffering. After we reassured her with an MRI (which we talk about in Chapter 7) of her brain that the headaches weren't the result of something harmful, her symptoms dissipated. Within two days, the patient was managing her headaches with non-prescription medicine. After taking stress-management training over the next few weeks, her headaches disappeared.

Applying the gate control theory to your experiences of pain can be a powerful tool for managing and relieving back pain. Allowing negative emotions such as anger, anxiety, frustration, hopelessness, and helplessness to overwhelm you can fling your pain gates wide open. Focusing on your pain, having no outside interests, worrying about the pain, and thinking you have no future all greatly increase your pain.

Conversely, increasing your activity, using short-term pain medication, exercising aerobically, and relaxing can make your pain gates close. Combine those tactics with positive thinking to distract you from the pain and you may be well on your way to recovery.

Understanding Categories of Pain

Understanding how pain is defined is important so you can find out how you can better control it. Health care professionals and researchers separate pain into three categories, each with different treatment approaches:

- **Acute pain:** This sort of pain lasts less than a month or is related directly to tissue damage or injury. Acute pain is the kind of pain you experience from a whiplash injury resulting from a car accident.

✔ **Chronic pain:** This pain is generally described as pain that lasts more than three to six months, or beyond the point of tissue healing. Chronic pain is usually less directly related to tissue damage or injury. Examples of chronic pain problems include long-term back pain and headaches.

✔ **Recurrent acute pain:** This intermittent type of pain is an acute pain episode that occurs over and over again. Examples of recurrent acute pain include episodes of acute back or neck pain that come and go, the cramps and pain associated with menstruation, and migraine headaches.

As we discuss later in this chapter and in Chapter 13, the longer your back pain persists, the more susceptible the pain is to influences such as negative thoughts and emotions as well as physical inactivity.

Debating the Need to Diagnose: Helpful or Harmful?

Doctors are trained to give diagnoses and patients are conditioned to expect diagnoses. But when it comes to spinal pain, the medical system's need to diagnose can do more harm than good.

Often, the evidence that your doctor's diagnostic explanation is actually causing your pain is sparse. In trying to comply with the medical establishment's system of examination, diagnosis, and treatment, health care professionals often focus on a supposed abnormality, but often the abnormality has nothing to do with your pain.

Most patients with back or neck pain would rather hear the doctor say 'Your pain's due to a bulging disc' or 'Your spine's out of alignment' than 'I don't know what's causing your pain.' But in reality, many back and neck pain problems are never accurately diagnosed.

The need to diagnose can lead to incorrect and unnecessary treatment. In many cases, your back or neck pain improves regardless of whether you receive treatment.

Don't despair when your doctor can't make an exact diagnosis – only about 10–15 per cent of people with spinal pain ever find a specific diagnosis. Even if you don't know what's causing your pain you can get effective treatment. About 90 per cent of people with back or neck pain recover, most within a week or so. Just realising that an episode of spinal pain isn't unusual can be the first step on the road to recovery.

In this section, we discuss how the medical establishment diagnoses your condition and why the process can let down people with spinal pain. We also tackle emotional and psychological factors and their roles in back and neck pain.

Diagnosing based on an imaging scan

Doctors sometimes make a diagnosis based upon an imaging scan. Some practitioners believe that showing you an alleged 'problem' on an X-ray provides a diagnosis. What some doctors don't realise is that telling you these findings are significant can lead you to believe – wrongly – that your spine's damaged. In most cases, the findings on the scan have absolutely nothing to do with your pain.

Dr Sinel had an all-too-typical case: A 40-year-old patient had been told by another doctor that his lower back pain was due to arthritic changes seen on an X-ray. The patient thought that his spine had deteriorated so much at the age of 40 that he was experiencing back pain. He assumed that things were sure to get worse, even though the doctor didn't explicitly say so.

The truth is that you see arthritic changes on the X-rays of most 40-year-old men and women who don't have back or neck pain. So although the findings on your X-ray may have nothing to do with your pain, the doctor may pinpoint them as the source of your pain to satisfy the medical establishment's need for a diagnosis.

Recognising the role of psychological and emotional factors

Never underestimate the role of psychological and emotional factors in back and neck pain. Some doctors – including us – think that emotions and stress contribute to and prolong a great deal of back and neck pain. In common conditions such as stress-related back or neck pain and chronic back and neck pain syndrome (we discuss both of these later in this chapter), psychological factors play a key role in exacerbating and extending the pain.

If your practitioner isn't aware of emotional influences on spinal pain, the likelihood of an incorrect diagnosis and inappropriate treatment increases. If you think that emotional factors may be a part of your back or neck pain, discuss these factors with your doctor. Don't be deterred if your doctor discounts the possibility – keep searching until you find a doctor who treats you as a whole person, both mind and body.

Understanding the Deconditioning Syndrome

The *deconditioning* or *deactivation syndrome* occurs when you try to alleviate your back or neck pain by limiting normal activities, restricting exercise, or resting more. The deconditioning syndrome can be part of any of the diagnoses that we discuss later in this chapter.

The deconditioning syndrome begins when you avoid activity – often on the recommendation of a health care professional or because you discover less activity initially causes you less pain. Rather than helping you, inactivity may make a bad situation worse. By reducing your activities, you eventually decrease the size, strength, and flexibility of your muscles and ligaments, as well as your cardiovascular and muscular endurance.

If you're experiencing the deconditioning syndrome, getting active again to strengthen those muscles is important. Your spinal pain is unlikely to be harmful, even though it hurts. We strongly encourage you to resume normal activities as soon as possible. Chapter 15 suggests loads of ways to exercise your way back to health.

Considering Conditions That Cause Spinal Pain

Spinal pain is notoriously difficult to diagnose: The cause is rarely just physical, in the way that a broken leg has a clear-cut physical cause. Because of the close relationship between your mind and body in general – and your mind and back in particular – psychological factors strongly influence back and neck pain. Various emotional, mental, and physical factors can cause back pain, as shown in Figure 3-2.

Herniated disc . . . pinched nerve . . . bulging disc. You've probably heard all these diagnoses before – and you may feel unnecessarily anxious about them. But fear not: Most diagnoses for back and neck pain aren't as awful as they sound. In this section, we look at the full range of conditions – common and rare – that cause back and neck pain. For each condition, we look at the symptoms, the diagnosis, the treatment options, and the outlook for recovery.

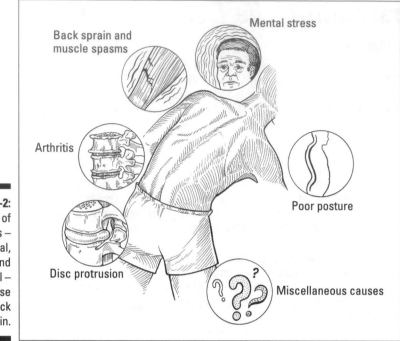

Figure 3-2:
A variety of
influences —
physical,
mental, and
emotional —
can cause
your back
pain.

A few very rare but serious conditions — cauda equina syndrome, spinal tumour, and spinal infection — require aggressive medical treatment. Your doctor can diagnose these conditions quickly with modern testing techniques. These conditions often require surgery, and we discuss them more fully in Chapter 9.

Herniated disc/arm pain/sciatica

Your spinal discs lie between your vertebrae (the bones of your back) and act as cushions for the spine. A disc bulge or herniation occurs when the inner part of the disc, which is soft and gel-like, pushes out between the vertebrae. This problem can arise in one of two ways:

- **Bulging disc:** This condition occurs when the fluid inside a disc bulges out but doesn't actually break through the disc wall. Figure 3-3 shows a bulging disc. Bulging discs are commonly seen on MRI scans (which we talk about in Chapter 7). Bulging discs don't usually cause any symptoms because the nerve roots of the spine aren't irritated or compressed.

- **Herniated disc:** This condition occurs when the fluid inside a disc bulges towards the back of your body and breaks through the outer ring of the disc wall called the *annulus fibrosis* (see Figure 3-4).

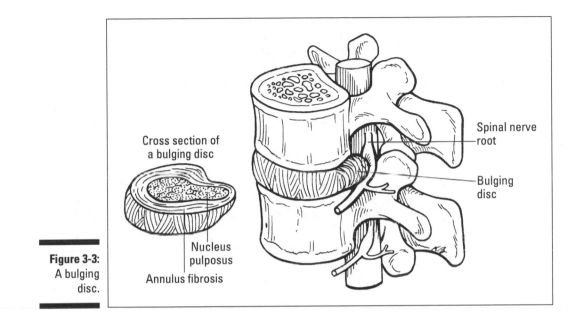

Cross section of
a bulging disc

Spinal nerve
root

Bulging
disc

Nucleus
pulposus

Annulus fibrosis

Figure 3-3:
A bulging
disc.

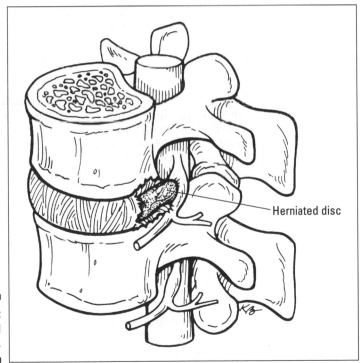

Herniated disc

Figure 3-4:
A herniated
disc.

When a disc is herniated, the disc material that has moved out of its usual space may press against a nearby spinal nerve, which may irritate it and may produce pain. *Sciatica* is commonly called a pinched nerve, but this is not always the case. Sciatica can occur when a herniated disc compresses the nerves of your lumbar spine (lower back). Because these nerves supply the sensation and strength to your legs and feet, a disc problem in your lower back can cause symptoms in your legs, such as weakness or numbness. (Note that you can also have sciatica when a nerve is irritated but not compressed.)

Sciatic pain has the following characteristics:

- More than 90 per cent of lumbar herniated discs occur between the last two levels of the lower spine (between L4 and L5 and between L5 and S1). Check out Figures 2-1 and 2-7 in Chapter 2 to see a picture of the lower spine.

- Sciatic pain typically occurs in the buttocks, the back of the thigh, and the calf, and occasionally down to the foot and heel.

- A disc herniation usually compresses but doesn't compromise the nerve as the nerve leaves your back and goes down your leg (Figure 3-5 shows how a herniated disc compresses against a nerve). The nerve is irritated, but still works. Occasionally, however, the nerve is so compressed that it causes a decrease in strength, feeling, and reflex. In this case, you may need surgery (which we talk about in Chapter 9).

If your doctor thinks you have a disc herniation, the following checklist can help you get a proper diagnosis:

- **Be sure that your doctor gives you a full physical examination.** This thorough examination should include looking at your neck, arms, hips, thighs, legs, and feet, testing how your nerves are working in these areas, and strength-testing all the individual muscle groups of the arms and legs. A good physical examination tells the doctor whether you have a disc problem and which nerve roots are affected. Based upon the physical examination, your doctor can determine whether you need any high-tech imaging studies (which we talk about in Chapter 7).

- **Remember that you don't always need sophisticated tests such as an MRI scan, even if your doctor suspects you have a herniated disc.** In most cases, your practitioner can diagnose and treat your herniated disc and sciatica successfully without any imaging studies. Generally, you need these studies only if your condition gets worse or you consider surgical treatment.

- **Don't accept a diagnosis of a herniated disc as the cause of your pain based simply on an MRI scan.** Even if your MRI scan shows a herniated disc, your doctor should still give you a careful physical examination. Your doctor should determine a high correlation between your symptoms and the location of the disc herniation; otherwise the MRI findings may mean absolutely nothing.

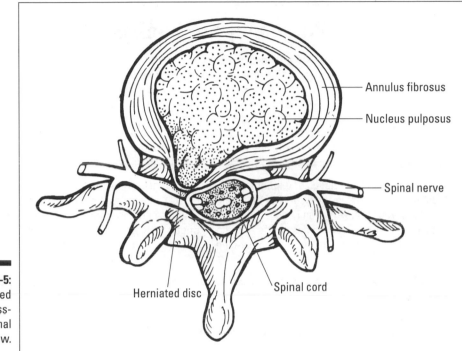

Annulus fibrosus

Nucleus pulposus

Spinal nerve

Spinal cord

Herniated disc

Figure 3-5:
Herniated
disc cross-
sectional
view.

If you've had symptoms of a disc herniation for less than a month, your doctor may recommend conservative treatment such as physiotherapy, exercises, and anti-inflammatory medication or epidural steroid injections to reduce any swelling. You may find some complementary medicine procedures, such as yoga, acupuncture, and massage useful (peruse Part III for more on complementary medicine).

The natural healing pattern of a disc herniation is favourable. Most herniated discs can be treated using non-surgical conservative management such as a combination of physiotherapy, exercises, medication, and healing time (which we discuss in Chapter 8). Most people get better within two to three months of conservative treatment. Don't panic about mild sensory loss, reflex loss, or weakness associated with a herniated disc: These functions usually return to normal as you recover.

Even if your symptoms last more than three months, you can still continue conservative management. Ongoing pain and symptoms are not necessarily reasons to have surgery, and you may improve even after three months. Your doctor may recommend surgery, but don't assume surgery's your only option. Surgical decisions should be based on very specific rules, which we discuss in Chapter 9.

Pregnancy and back pain

One of the more common side effects of pregnancy is back pain. Some women describe the back pain as 'discomfort', but others find the pain almost unbearable. If you have a history of back pain, you may be concerned about how pregnancy may affect your pain. Thankfully, you can manage your back pain effectively as you go through your pregnancy.

As your abdominal muscles expand during pregnancy, the muscles lose some of their ability to keep your spine erect and stable. This lack of stability and changes in your centre of gravity can cause your posture to change, leading to back pain.

You can do a few things to prevent or minimise back pain during pregnancy. Pay attention to your posture as much as possible (see Chapter 14 for details). You may also find a specialised yoga class for pregnancy an excellent way to ease your back pain. Always check with your doctor before beginning any exercise programme during pregnancy.

Inadequate calcium in your diet can cause muscle spasms. You may require more calcium when you're pregnant and/or breastfeeding. Check with your doctor to determine whether you're getting adequate calcium.

The sprain–strain diagnosis

A *sprain–strain injury* is a common diagnosis used in the medical treatment of spinal pain. This diagnosis has a great number of definitions. A sprain–strain is an injury to the muscles, ligaments, or tendons of the spine caused by an injury (due to a sports activity or lifting a heavy object, for example), poor posture, or lack of physical conditioning over time (or a combination of these problems).

A sprain–strain isn't serious and usually heals just like any other injury. Following an exercise and conditioning programme helps prevent sprain–strain injuries from recurring. You may be tempted to spend a few days in bed with a back injury, but remember that resting for any longer than that is one of the worst things you can do for a sprain–strain injury.

Typical symptoms of a sprain–strain injury include the following:

- **Pain, tightness, and spasms in your neck, shoulders, or lower back:** Pain may occur quickly, such as in response to an injury, or build up slowly over time, when you can't identify any specific injury.

- **Tenderness:** The muscles on either side of your spine and down to the upper part of your buttock area may be more sensitive than usual.

✔ **Pain that worsens on turning your head, or by bending forward or to the sides:** In severe cases, this pain may be associated with a muscle spasm.

✔ **Pain that's worse in the morning and then improves with activity over the course of the day:** This pattern is common in sprain–strain injuries – the muscles seem to warm up and the discomfort subsides as you move around.

No specific test exists for a sprain–strain injury. The diagnosis is usually based upon history and the absence of other findings that suggest any type of nerve root irritation.

Some doctors link sprain–strain to some type of activity associated with the onset of the injury, but we try to avoid doing this. If a practitioner pinpoints certain activities as the cause of your pain, you may develop a fear about these movements. We've seen patients with serious fears of making almost any movement: They limit their activities and soon develop a full-blown case of the deconditioning syndrome (which we talk about earlier in this chapter).

In most cases of sprain–strain, following a simple treatment programme alleviates your symptoms and returns you to full functioning activities. Try the following:

✔ Stop or reduce temporarily any activity that increases your symptoms, but try to maintain some level of activity. Then gradually increase your activity over several weeks.

✔ Put ice on the painful areas during the first 24–48 hours after injury. To avoid burning your skin, limit your ice use to 20 minutes every two hours. Don't put the ice in direct contact with your skin; instead, wrap it in a cold, wet tea towel.

✔ Take paracetamol or a non-steroidal anti-inflammatory medication to ease the pain (check out Chapter 6 for more on painkilling drugs).

✔ Rest in bed for a couple of days if you feel you must.

✔ Take muscle relaxants (such as Valium or Robaxin on prescription) for three to four days if your injury's severe.

✔ Resume your normal activities gradually. Try some light stretching and movement on the third or fourth day to prevent you becoming fearful of movement and to keep your muscles conditioned.

In some cases – for example, if you've developed a fear of re-injury – you may find additional formal treatment necessary for sprain–strain injury. Physiotherapy can help by supporting and guiding your return to activity as well as reducing acute pain and spasm.

Cervical migraine and headaches

Some experts think migraine's a very common misdiagnosis in general practice. Many doctors diagnose migraine when a person's headaches are recurrent, unilateral, and described as radiating from the back of the skull to the forehead or eye. However, if your doctor diagnoses you with migraine, consider having your neck examined by an osteopath, chiropractor, or a relevant medical specialist. Cervical (neck) problems cause a third of all headaches.

The whiplash neck

Whiplash neck is a very common sequel to a car accident in which your neck is jolted. Neck pain is a common symptom of whiplash neck and is usually correctly diagnosed as coming from the cervical spine. Headache is also a common consequence of a traffic accident, but many doctors miss the connection between headache and whiplash neck; instead, many doctors diagnose people with headache after a car crash as depressed or having a post-traumatic neurosis and put them on antidepressants or other drugs – but the treatment is unsuccessful in treating the headache. If you have a headache following a car accident, get your cervical spine checked out by an osteopath, chiropractor, or a relevant medical specialist.

Bizarre (ear, nose, and throat) neck symptoms

Neck problems can cause bizarre symptoms, including dizziness, pallor, sweating, nausea, and ringing in the ears. These symptoms often follow an accident or fall. If you have symptoms such as these, but your practitioner finds no ear, nose, or throat cause, ask your practitioner to look at your neck: Treatment to the neck under these circumstances is often successful, but it is likely that treatment directed elsewhere, if the neck is the cause, won't help.

Neck, shoulder, and arm pain

The neck's a common source of arm pain, so if you have arm pain your doctor should examine your neck. If your doctor isn't interested in your neck, consider getting a second opinion (ask your GP for a referral). The cervical spine can cause symptoms and signs that mimic local arm conditions, and your practitioner may misdiagnose such symptoms as, for example, tennis elbow. Local treatment to the arm in these circumstances achieves nothing.

Stress-related back and neck pain

Stress-related back and neck pain isn't a conventional medical diagnosis. But based on our experience, we believe stress is a common cause of back and neck pain. Typical symptoms include diffuse muscle aches (including back or neck pain), sleep disturbance, depression, anxiety, and fatigue.

Because many conventional medical doctors aren't familiar with the diagnosis of stress-related back and neck pain, you may have to raise the possibility yourself if you think that stress is causing your pain. As in a sprain–strain injury, stress-related back and neck pain is diagnosed based on your history and an absence of structural causes of pain such as a herniated disc.

Most people with spinal pain focus on the physical problem. If your back or neck pain is stress-related, looking at the emotional issues is essential for improvement. Part of your treatment for this condition may include psychotherapy or stress counselling to help you take control of the emotional issues causing your pain. We often recommend that our patients 'think psychological, not physical' when the pain occurs. A physiotherapist can reassure you as you increase your activities and challenge your pain.

Arthritis of the spine

Arthritis is a general term meaning inflammation of a joint or joints in any part of your body, including the spine. Arthritis has many different causes and comes in many types. Some types of arthritis are part of the natural ageing process and cause no pain, but other types cause severe deformation of the joints and pain.

Many people associate the term 'arthritis' with rheumatoid arthritis, which causes pain and malformation of joints in the body. The good news is that rheumatoid arthritis rarely affects the spine. When discussing arthritis of the spine, doctors usually refer to findings on X-rays and MRI scans that are part of the natural ageing process. Arthritic changes in joints occur naturally with age and don't produce pain symptoms themselves.

The term 'arthritis' should rarely be used when discussing joint changes in the spine. We frequently see young and middle-aged patients saying things like 'My doctor told me I have the spine of an 80-year-old.' A message like this causes great suffering and fear for no reason.

Psychosomatic pain: not just in your head

When emotional issues are thought to cause physical problems, the condition is described as *psychosomatic* or *psycho-physiological*. People generally think – mistakenly – that psychosomatic medical conditions are imaginary. In fact *psychosomatic* means that an emotional issue has caused a real physical problem.

Psychosomatic conditions include certain types of asthma, neck pain, headaches, ulcers, skin problems, and back pain. No one would argue that these aren't real physical medical problems: They cause very real stress, discomfort, pain, and disability.

Simple changes in your lifestyle can go a long way to preventing and treating your psychosomatic back pain. The first step towards making a full recovery is to work with a physiotherapist who can help you identify the source of your psychosomatic pain and provide support and encouragement as you work through the pain.

Degenerative disc disease

In degenerative disc disease, the soft central portion of the disc loses some of its water content and begins to dry out. The first image in Figure 3-6 shows a normal disc; the second image shows that disc degeneration has occurred, which decreases the disc's height, narrows the *foramen* (or opening), and misaligns the facet joint.

Think of degenerative disc disease as being similar to getting grey hair: The condition isn't really a disease at all but a term that describes the wear and tear of normal ageing. Degenerative disc disease is simply a part of the ageing process, and everyone is affected to varying degrees.

Sometimes degenerative disc disease leads to a mechanical type of low back pain if you're not physically fit and attempt strenuous activity. Degenerative disc disease is treated with appropriate exercise, and anti-inflammatory medication. The disease rarely requires surgical treatment.

Facet syndrome

A *facet joint* is a joint between two vertebrae. Facet joints allow your vertebrae to move while keeping your spine in proper alignment. Like all joints, facet joints are subject to wear and tear and begin to change as you get older. If you have *facet syndrome*, you have an inflammation of one or more of your facet joints. Inflammation of these joints can produce *referred pain* – that is, pain that you feel in a place other than where the pain is being caused.

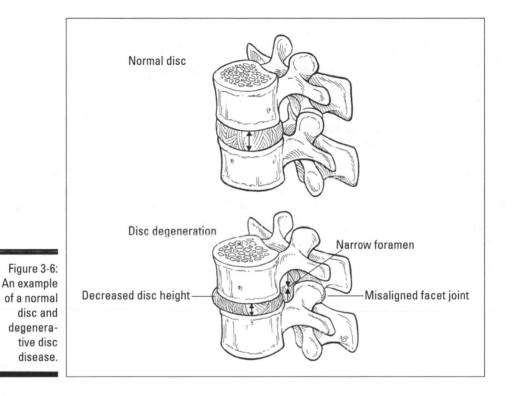

Figure 3-6:
An example
of a normal
disc and
degenera-
tive disc
disease.

Facet syndrome may cause tenderness in an area about 4 centimetres to the side of your spine in your upper or lower back. Pressure in your lower back may cause discomfort and sometimes pain down into your buttock or thigh area. You may notice that the pain gets worse when you bend sideways or backwards, twist your waist, or stand on one leg.

Facet syndrome isn't serious. The problem can be painful, but the pain usually goes away within two to three weeks. Treatment of facet syndrome is the same as for a sprain–strain injury: Temporarily stop or reduce any activity that worsens your symptoms; apply ice to the painful areas for the first 24–48 hours after injury; take anti-inflammatory medication; use a back brace or collar to reduce movement; and gradually resume normal activities and movement. If facet syndrome becomes chronic, your practitioner may suggest you have an injection into the irritated joint of a *facet block*, an anti-inflammatory and anaesthetic medication.

High anxiety: a new theory about stress-related back pain

Dr John Sarno, of New York University's Medical Center, popularised the notion of stress-related back pain in several books. He believes that a person's emotions – especially pent-up anger and anxiety, which have serious negative effects on the body – cause stress-related back pain. We work with Dr Sarno and have witnessed some dramatic results.

Dr Sarno suggests that certain personality types are more likely than others to get stress-related back pain. According to Dr Sarno, the following personality characteristics interact with stressful life situations to cause stress-related back pain:

✔ Being driven strongly to succeed

✔ Holding a strong sense of responsibility

✔ Being self-motivated and disciplined

✔ Being harshly critical of yourself

✔ Having perfectionist and compulsive tendencies

Dr Sarno believes that your mind, when faced with a stressful emotional situation, may push emotional tension and stress out of your awareness and into your unconscious. This unconscious tension from emotional stress causes muscle tension, spasm, and pain in your lower back and elsewhere. Your mind chooses the distraction of physical pain instead of dealing with the actual emotional issues that your mind perceives as more threatening.

Awareness and understanding of how your mind can deal with emotional stress is the first step toward healing stress-related back pain. Dr Sarno warns against repressing your anger or emotions and says you shouldn't let back pain intimidate you. He also says not to think of yourself as injured, because psychological conditioning can contribute to ongoing back pain.

Dr Sarno suggests resuming physical activity, telling your brain you won't be intimidated by pain any more, and stopping all treatments for your back, as they may be blocking your recovery.

Arachnoiditis

Arachnoiditis is scarring of the connective tissue (the spinal arachnoid) around your spinal nerve roots. *Arachnoid* literally means 'like a cobweb' and describes what the condition looks like on imaging studies. The most common cause of arachnoiditis is previous surgery in the affected area. Symptoms include pain, numbness, and tingling in your legs – but you may have no symptoms at all, despite an MRI scan showing you have arachnoiditis. Arachnoiditis can be difficult to treat because its symptoms are not very responsive to conventional treatments for back and neck pain. Your doctor may prescribe painkillers or a cortisone injection. If you have severe arachnoiditis, your practitioner may recommend a spinal cord stimulator (for more on spinal cord stimulators, check out Chapter 7).

Surgeons often avoid performing spinal surgery if arachnoiditis is present, because surgery can make the condition worse. If you have arachnoiditis, proceed very cautiously. Surgery cannot treat arachnoiditis and may actually make the problem worse.

Check out www.arachnoiditis.co.uk for more information.

Spondylolisthesis and spondylolysis

Spondylolisthesis literally means 'slipping vertebrae' and describes a condition in which one of your vertebrae slips over another (see Figure 3-7). The cause is often a fracture or crack (called a *spondylolysis*) in part of the vertebrae, which may be due to changes related to ageing (known as *degenerative changes*) or repetitive overstrain.

Figure 3-7:
Notice how the two vertebrae are slipping (spondylolisthesis) due to the fracture (spondylolysis).

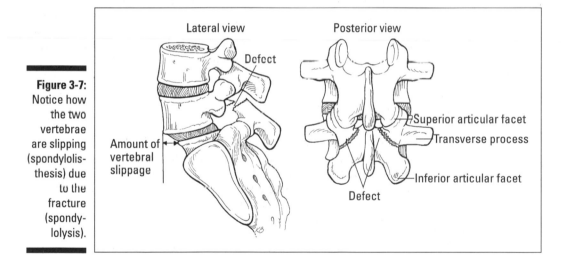

A spondylolysis often results from trauma occurring over a period of time during your teenage years. Sports and activities that involve repeated *hyperextension* (bending over backwards) are often the culprit. Although you can get spondylolisthesis for many reasons, both in childhood and adulthood, the condition is most common in gymnasts, ballet dancers, and football players. Typically, a single episode of hyperextension does not cause a problem, but repeated episodes can result in an actual break.

Spondylolisthesis can cause pain in the lower back and, occasionally, sciatic pain if the nerve roots are involved. A very common indicator of spondylolisthesis in a young person is backache that lasts for more than a couple of weeks.

If your doctor suspects you have this condition, you should have a bone scan, which can detect very fine fractures in your vertebrae. (We discuss bone scans in Chapter 7.) If the problem is diagnosed at the time the fracture occurs (usually between the ages of 13 and 16 years), the condition can be treated effectively and completely. Treatment usually includes a brace and restriction of activities for about four months to allow the fracture to heal. In severe cases of slipping, spinal fusion surgery in which two adjacent vertebrae are fused together maybe necessary. We discuss fusion surgery in Chapter 9. If this condition goes undiagnosed when it occurs in childhood, the result can be back problems later in life.

The other common type of spondylolisthesis is called *degenerative spondylolisthesis*. This condition is caused by severe wear-and-tear changes in the facet joints or connecting joints of your lower back due to a variety of reasons. The most common location for this condition is between the fourth and fifth lumbar vertebrae, with the fourth vertebra slipping forwards (towards your stomach) over the fifth vertebra. Treatment is the same as for spondylolisthesis.

Coccydynia

Coccydynia literally means pain in the *coccyx*, the tailbone at the bottom of your spine. Coccydynia occurs most often as a result of trauma, usually a direct fall on the buttocks, which can break your tailbone. However, you may have pain near your coccyx for no known reason. Coccydynia can also cause persistent pain and tenderness just above your rectal area – the condition can be a real pain in the bum! Coccydynia is often diagnosed simply by the symptoms: In many cases, nothing unusual is seen on X-rays. Diagnosis is based on physical examination, history of pain in the coccyx area with or without trauma, and sometimes X-rays.

If you have coccydynia, you can expect the treatment to include several things. First, the painfully obvious: Avoid sitting on hard surfaces. Try using a doughnut-shaped cushion to control your pain when sitting down. If you have more resistant pain, your practitioner may suggest anti-inflammatory medication or a local injection of anaesthetic and cortisone. Recent research suggests that a special type of biofeedback (which we talk about in Chapter 13) that shows you how to relax local muscle spasm can also help.

You may consider surgery to remove the coccyx as a last resort if you have severe chronic coccydynia. However, we've seen many people who've had surgery, only to find that their pain continues. To find out more about coccydynia surgery, head to Chapter 9.

Spinal fractures

Spinal fractures, diagnosed with X-rays, are almost always caused by one of the following:

- ✔ A severe trauma such as a road traffic accident or fall
- ✔ A disease that weakens the spinal bones, such as osteoporosis and cancer of the spine

Typical warning signs of a possible spinal fracture include the following:

- ✔ Pain occurring suddenly in middle-aged or elderly persons after bending or lifting
- ✔ Pain that worsens with activity
- ✔ Pain so severe that it wakes you up at night
- ✔ Pain that doesn't go away within a week or two

If you suspect you have a spinal fracture, see a doctor familiar with spinal problems immediately.

An X-ray can detect a fracture. *Compression fractures*, which are more common in people with diseases that weaken the spinal bones, are easily detected through an X-ray because these fractures often cause a characteristic appearance to the *vertebral body*, the large front part of the vertebrae that's cushioned by the discs (refer to Chapter 2).

Treatment includes strong or codeine/morphine based painkillers for the first two to three weeks. You may need to take long-term narcotic painkillers, restrict your activity, and use a brace for up to three months as the fracture heals. The prognosis is excellent, and your fracture is likely to heal and allow you to return to normal activities.

Subluxation

Subluxation, or a limitation of movement in a joint, is a term frequently used by chiropractors to explain the cause of lower back pain. Various chiropractic treatments are used to restore a joint that is supposedly subluxed or restricted. This diagnosis is controversial among physicians who treat spinal problems. Not all doctors are convinced that subluxed joints actually exist and cause pain. We discuss chiropractic treatment in Chapter 11.

Lumbar spinal stenosis

Lumbar spinal stenosis is a narrowing of the spinal canal that causes a compression or pinching of the nerves that go to the buttocks and legs. Stenosis can result from any of the following:

- Disc bulges
- Wear-and-tear changes that create bony spurs
- Overgrowth of the facet joint
- Congenital (meaning 'present from birth') narrowing of the spinal canal

Lumbar spinal stenosis usually presents with pain in the buttocks and legs that

- Limits your ability to walk for any great distance or at a fast pace
- Goes away if you lean forwards at the waist as you walk – for example, you may get relief by leaning on your shopping trolley in the supermarket
- Relieves if you sit down for a short period of time or until your symptoms subside

Diagnosis of lumbar spinal stenosis is based on your medical history, a physical examination, and imaging studies. This condition is seen more frequently after the age of 65, due to ageing of the spine.

Lumbar stenosis tends to worsen over time, but it doesn't lead to paralysis, shorten your life, or kill you. The most common consequences are limitations in your activities. Usually, the symptoms progress slowly. Sometimes, the condition improves, even though your MRI scans look worse – but nobody knows why.

Treatment for lumbar spinal stenosis consists of three phases:

1. Your doctor, depending on your symptoms, may recommend an exercise programme combined with anti-inflammatory drugs.

2. Your doctor may recommend you have an epidural steroid injection into the space surrounding the spinal nerves. This often provides dramatic relief and may last for several years before you need another injection.

3. Your practitioner may suggest surgical widening of your spinal canal. This procedure involves a *laminectomy*, or removal of the bony part of each vertebra (see Chapter 2 for the anatomical details). Remember that undergoing surgery for this condition is your decision to make, depending on your tolerance of the symptoms and your quality of life. Check out Chapter 9 for more on spinal surgery.

Chronic back and neck pain syndrome

Chronic back and neck pain syndrome is a group of symptoms that occur when your pain lasts for more than about three to six months – beyond the point of tissue healing (see Figure 3-8). This syndrome goes beyond simple physical deconditioning, which we discuss earlier in this chapter. Both physical and mental deconditioning can cause chronic back and neck pain syndrome: If you don't use 'em, you lose 'em.

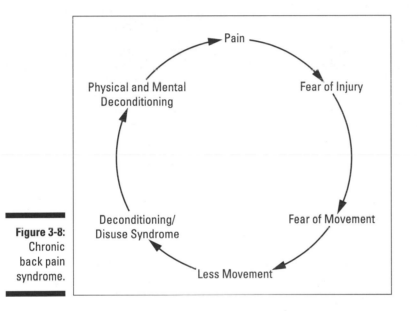

Figure 3-8:
Chronic back pain syndrome.

Research shows that the physical findings in people with chronic back or neck pain are no more serious than in people whose back or neck injury heals in the normal amount of time. We believe stress and other emotional factors probably contribute to chronic pain. Changes in blood flow patterns to the spinal muscles and anxiety about the pain may keep the muscles perpetually in spasm. Over treating back and neck pain with rest and *passive therapy* (therapy that involves no activity on your part, such as applying heat and cold) can lead to deconditioning and the chronic pain syndrome.

Chronic back and neck pain syndrome often gets worse over time and includes physical and psychological symptoms. By the time the syndrome is fully developed, many of the symptoms aren't related to the original pain problem but are due to deconditioning, overuse of pain medication, depression, anxiety, and social isolation.

Failed back surgery syndrome

In our opinion, failed back surgery syndrome occurs most commonly when a person wrongly has spinal surgery. Unfortunately, failed back surgery syndrome is all too common. The symptoms are similar to chronic back pain syndrome, except that they arise after spine surgery. The following items can all lead to failed back surgery syndrome:

✔ Early infection after spinal surgery

✔ Spinal surgery carried out at the wrong level of the spine or that doesn't heal properly

✔ Psychological distress

✔ Inadequate rehabilitation reconditioning after spinal surgery

✔ Another structural problem, such as stenosis or arachnoiditis

The best treatment for failed back surgery syndrome is to avoid surgery in the first place. Be very wary of spinal surgery and make the decision to undergo it only after careful consideration of all the alternatives. We discuss spinal surgery in more detail in Chapter 9.

If you have failed back surgery syndrome, your further treatment should never consist of just more spinal surgery. Instead, try a conservative non-surgical approach similar to that used for chronic back pain syndrome. Focus on treating your physical, psychological, and emotional issues simultaneously.

If you have chronic back or neck pain syndrome, you probably need multidisciplinary treatment to treat all aspects of your problem simultaneously. Treatment may include the following:

✔ Physical exercise and reactivation to address your deconditioning

✔ Psychological intervention to address mental deconditioning and emotional issues

✔ Detoxification to address medication dependence and substance abuse problems (not an issue in all cases)

✔ Return to work or other activity that provides you with a sense of purpose

✔ Various medications including antidepressants, which are often prescribed as part of a comprehensive treatment programme

Exploring Other Conditions That Cause Back and Neck Pain

The conditions we describe here aren't usually the primary cause of significant back or neck pain. If you have one of these conditions, you may have some or no associated pain. We mention these diagnoses here because our patients often ask us about them.

Discitis

Discitis, or inflammation of the disc, is a rare condition. Although doctors don't know the exact cause of discitis, the condition may be caused by a bacterial or viral infection in the disc space. The result is inflammation and pain. You're more likely to develop discitis if you have diabetes or immune system problems. If bacteria have caused your discitis, your doctor is likely to prescribe antibiotics. In children, discitis may be treated with a back brace.

Fibromyalgia

If you have chronic spinal pain, sleep disturbance, multiple tender joints, fatigue, diffuse pain, and limitations of activity, your practitioner may diagnose you with *fibromyalgia*. This is an ill-defined condition that is the source of much discussion and debate.

If you have fibromyalgia, you may have other symptoms such as bowel problems, tingling and numbness, chronic headaches, chest pain, memory problems, anxiety, and depression. No medical test exists for diagnosing fibromyalgia.

Several terms have been used to describe fibromyalgia, including myofascial pain syndrome, myositis, fibrositis, and tension myalgia. Doctors don't understand what causes or cures fibromyalgia, but many treatments can help you.

Current treatment programmes generally include anti-inflammatory medications to relieve pain, antidepressant medications for their effect on sleep and depression, and a gradual increase in activities through appropriate exercise. You can also use various complementary medicine approaches (which we discuss in Part III) to augment this general treatment approach.

If you have fibromyalgia, choose your treatments carefully. People with fibromyalgia often go from one treatment to the next, searching for a cure. Sadly, they rarely get any real benefit.

We strongly believe that psychological and emotional issues are part of fibromyalgia. Whether these issues cause, or are a reaction to, fibromyalgia is unknown. One thing's clear: If you don't address your psychological and emotional issues as part of the treatment, your treatment's unlikely to be successful.

Consider the following treatments if you have fibromyalgia:

- ✔ Anti-inflammatory drugs for your pain

- ✔ Antidepressant medications to improve your sleep, relieve depression, and provide pain relief

- ✔ An exercise programme that gradually increases your activities and encourages you to return to a normal lifestyle

- ✔ Complementary medicine (see Part III for more info) to help you manage your symptoms and return to a normal life

- ✔ Paying attention to psychological and emotional issues that may increase your level of suffering, hamper your attempts at keeping a positive mental attitude, and prevent you from recovering

Osteomyelitis

Osteomyelitis is a rare infection in the vertebrae or bones of the spine. Symptoms include back or neck pain when resting, weight loss, and fever. A number of test results can detect osteomyelitis, including abnormal blood findings. Osteomyelitis is treated with a brace and appropriate antibiotics for three to six weeks.

Scoliosis

Scoliosis describes a curvature of the spine. Scoliosis, which occurs in several different varieties, rarely causes lower back pain in people under 40 years old, unless it's very severe. Watching out for scoliosis in young people, especially teenage girls, is important, because early treatment with a brace can help avoid surgery later on.

The key to managing scoliosis is determining whether it's progressive (curving more and more over time). A small percentage of people with scoliosis in the lower back have progressive disease that needs treatment with an exercise programme, brace, and possibly spinal surgery. However, most people diagnosed with scoliosis have no back pain or any symptoms, and the condition requires no specific treatment.

Scoliosis is commonly given as a reason for lower back pain with recommendations for extensive treatment to straighten out the spine. In these cases, your back pain may actually be due to a disc, sprain–strain, deconditioning, or stress-related problem. If you have a scoliosis curve less than 20 degrees – as in the majority of cases seen clinically – you probably don't need treatment.

Transitional vertebrae

A transitional vertebra is either one extra or one fewer lumbar vertebrae than normal and is often seen on X-rays. Transitional vertebrae are found at the base of the lumbar spine where it connects to the sacrum (refer to Figure 2-6 in Chapter 2 for more info). The condition isn't usually associated with low back pain. If you have a transitional vertebra, just consider yourself unique and ignore it.

Osteoporosis

Osteoporosis can weaken the bones of the spine, making them susceptible to spinal fractures. Elderly women are most likely to suffer from osteoporosis. If you experience pain from a fracture caused by osteoporosis, the fracture is usually minimal and lasts three to six weeks.

Treatment usually consists of limiting your activities, taking mild painkillers, and using an appropriate brace for your lower back. Your doctor should investigate the condition of osteoporosis that caused the weakening. Appropriate medications such as supplemental calcium or oestrogen therapy may be helpful.

Chapter 4

Finding Someone to Help with Back and Neck Pain

In This Chapter

▶ Understanding the medical community

▶ Knowing what questions to ask

▶ Getting safe alternative treatments

▶ Developing a positive relationship with your practitioner

As you search for relief from your back or neck pain, you may consult a variety of health care professionals. We don't have room in this book to list all the professionals who treat back and neck pain, but the common ones include general practitioners (GPs), osteopaths, orthopaedic surgeons, rheumatologists, physiotherapists, neurologists, neurosurgeons, and pain clinic consultants. Chiropractors, acupuncturists, and massage therapists are also involved in treating back and neck pain. All these different names can get confusing, so we explain the different professionals in this chapter. We also suggest some questions to ask the professionals treating you, so that you can work in partnership with your health care providers.

Who Treats Back and Neck Pain?

Finding your way through today's confusing medical culture is like visiting a foreign country where you don't speak the language or know the lay of the land. You may become scared and confused, especially if you don't have a map or dictionary. In this section, we lead you through the nomenclature so you don't end up being a bewildered tourist without a clue as to what's going on around you.

The UK medical community's arranged at two levels of specialisation:

✔ **Primary care:** GPs handle a variety of medical problems. These doctors have a good understanding of all aspects of medicine and often act as co-ordinators or managers of your treatment programme.

✔ **Secondary care:** Specialists in disciplines such as orthopaedics, neurology, neurosurgery, rheumatology, and pain clinics provide a more detailed evaluation of your back or neck pain along with more specific treatment approaches. These specialists see patients with all sorts of problems that fall within their area of expertise, including people with back and neck pain. For example, an orthopaedic surgeon treats a variety of orthopaedic problems, such as knee, elbow, and hip disorders, as well as back and neck pain.

Primary care doctors

General practitioners are often called *primary care physicians*. Your GP is usually the first person you consult for any type of medical problem, including back and neck pain. GPs are usually comfortable and confident treating a variety of medical problems, including back and neck pain.

When you see your GP because of back or neck pain, he or she checks whether anything's seriously wrong with your spine. If your GP finds no serious spinal disorder, he or she will probably treat you over the next six to eight weeks. If other symptoms occur or if your pain lingers, your doctor may refer you to a specialist. If your primary care doctor has been treating your back or neck pain for more than a few weeks and you're not getting any better, ask your doctor to refer you to a specialist.

Specialists

Orthopaedic surgeons, neurosurgeons, neurologists, rheumatologists, and pain clinic consultants are the medical specialists most likely to evaluate and treat your back or neck pain at the specialist level. Specialists in these areas may or may not focus on back and neck pain and spinal disorders. These specialists have followed a set programme of training for seven or eight years after qualifying in medicine and have postgraduate qualifications in their specialties. Here are a few brief definitions:

✔ Orthopaedic surgeons are consultants specialising in the surgery of the musculo-skeletal system.

✔ Neurosurgeons are consultant surgeons who specialise in treating the nervous system.

✔ Neurologists are consultant physicians who have advanced training in problems of the nervous system. They use non-surgical treatments.

✔ Rheumatologists are consultant physicians who specialise in arthritic problems.

Pain clinic consultants

Pain clinics – a relatively recent development – bring together a range of specialists to advise patients on the management of chronic pain, including back and neck pain. Consultant anaesthetists run most pain clinics because anaesthetists have a special interest in relieving pain. Other professionals involved may include psychologists, counsellors, and physiotherapists who combine their skills to help treat pain.

Unless you're admitted as an emergency patient through the Accident and Emergency department, the only way to see a consultant on the NHS (National Health Service) is with a referral from your GP. If you have any doubts or questions, discuss them with your GP. We show you how to find out more about your consultant in the section 'How Well Qualified Is Your Specialist?'.

Physiotherapists

Physiotherapists are autonomous practitioners who are fully trained to assess patients, diagnose, treat, and refer you back to your GP for further referral if necessary. Your GP or specialist may refer you to the physiotherapy department at your local hospital. Physiotherapists offer various treatments, including hot and cold therapies, traction, manipulation, and advice and instructions on exercises. Head to Chapter 8 for more on hot and cold treatments and traction, and see Chapter 15 for the low-down on exercise.

How Well Qualified Is Your Specialist?

You may want to know about your specialist's qualifications and particular medical interests. Medical practitioners must be registered with the General Medical Council (GMC) to work in the UK. To check that your doctor is GMC-registered, have a look at the Medical Register online at http://www.gmc-uk.org/register/search/index.asp.

You can also consult the Medical Directory, which provides contact details and brief biographies of around 140,000 medical practitioners who are resident in the UK. You can find the Medical Directory in most public lending libraries. It lists only medically qualified doctors. The directory tells you:

- ✔ The degrees and qualifications, place of training, and date of qualification of your consultant
- ✔ The postgraduate qualifications held by your consultant
- ✔ The medical and professional societies to which your consultant belongs
- ✔ The junior hospital posts that your consultant has held
- ✔ The current post held by your consultant and his or her speciality

If you need more info, try asking your GP or specialist. Nowadays, most medical practitioners agree that patients should be as fully informed as they want to be about their problems and treatment.

Dealing with Osteopaths, Chiropractors, and Other Complementary Practitioners

Osteopaths, chiropractors, acupuncturists, aromatherapists, and a whole host of other complementary practitioners treat many people with back and neck pain. This treatment may be primary (meaning that it replaces GP treatment) or in addition to standard medical care. In this section, we show you how to find out about these treatments in an informed manner.

Address the following issues before you obtain complementary medical care for your back or neck pain:

- ✔ **See your GP first:** Ask your doctor to evaluate your back or neck pain before you obtain complementary care. Your GP can rule out any serious causes of your pain, such as a tumour or infection. Your GP can also determine whether other treatments are safe for you.

- ✔ **Get a referral from a dependable source:** To investigate a referral, gather information from an appropriate professional society. You may also get referrals from family and friends who've had positive experiences with a particular treatment or practitioner. Remember to ask about the nature of the treatment and the outcome.

✔ **Ask questions:** When you first talk with a complementary medical practitioner, ask the following sorts of question:

- **Do you treat primarily back and neck pain problems?** You want to be sure that your practitioner is qualified to treat back and neck pain and treats patients with problems similar to yours frequently.

- **Can you work with my medical doctor?** Your complementary practitioner needs to be willing to work and communicate with your GP. Although communication may not always be necessary, you want to know that your practitioner is happy to talk to your physician or co-ordinate care if you, your physician, or practitioner feels it necessary.

- **Can you recommend exercises and other things I can do at home?** You need to know whether your complementary practitioner can suggest things to do on your own to help with your pain.

- **Can you tell me how long and how often I can expect to be treated?** Try to get an idea of how long and how often you need treatment, based on the practitioner's work with patients with problems similar to yours.

The warning signs of poor practice: Watch out!

You are more likely to find the following signs of poor practice in the complementary medicine arena. However, be concerned if *any* doctor

✔ Doesn't complete a history and clinical examination before beginning treatment

✔ Tries to get other members of your family to begin treatment

✔ Promises to prevent back or neck pain or disease through regular check-ups or manipulation

✔ Discourages you from getting a second opinion

If you have queries or concerns about practitioners and their qualifications you can contact:

Chiropractors

✔ The British Chiropractic Association, tel: 0118 950 5950, Web site www.chiropractic-uk.co.uk

✔ The General Chiropractic Council, tel: 0207 713 5155, Web site www.opsi.gov.uk

Osteopaths

✔ The British Osteopathic Association, tel: 01582 488 455, Web site www.applegate.co.uk

✔ The General Osteopathic Council, tel 0207 357 6655, Web site www.osteopathy.org.uk

In Appendix B we list other organisations that you may encounter in the world of complementary medicine so that you can obtain as much information as you need.

Building a Positive Relationship with Your Health Care Provider

Your relationship with the practitioner treating your back or neck pain problem is critical to you getting better. Significant problems with treatment can occur if the expectations of you and your doctor don't match. You may expect your practitioner to simply diagnose your problem and then fix it – but being a passive patient can have negative results. For instance, if your practitioner gives you an exercise programme but you don't follow it properly, the programme's unlikely to work.

Your back and neck pain treatment is likely to be most effective if you and your practitioner take an active role in seeking solutions. You may find being active in your treatment challenging because you find your practitioner intimidating. Some practitioners are uncomfortable with patients who want to be fully involved in their own treatment, perhaps thinking that the patient is questioning their judgement rather than trying to get the best care possible. If your practitioner is defensive when you ask questions, use the tips in Chapter 24 to help you work together successfully.

Chapter 5

Knowing Your Rights and Benefits

. . . .

In This Chapter

▶ Knowing your rights

▶ Exploring the alternatives

▶ Getting around the benefits jungle

▶ Finding out where to seek advice

. . . .

*O*ne of the main problems you may have as a person with back or neck pain is knowing what your rights are and what benefits you're entitled to. Many people with back and neck pain need information about taking time off work and their rights as a patient during treatment.

Negotiating the state benefits jungle is even more complicated. Each person's situation is different, and the mass of information that's available changes frequently. Knowing where to go for the right advice for your situation can be confusing.

Being Aware of Your Rights

To make the most of the help available, you need to be aware of your rights and benefits. Great efforts have been made over the years to emphasise patients' rights and increase their role in medical treatment.

These days you're actively encouraged to ask questions so that you have no doubts or uncertainties. As a patient, you should feel reassured and confident that you're getting the best treatment for your situation – and clinicians are urged to make sure that you do.

You have the right to ask your practitioner to explain clearly any proposed treatment, including any risks involved and any alternatives, before you decide whether to have the treatment.

NHS complaints procedures

Unfortunately, sometimes things go wrong. Always approach the practitioner and his or her manager first before things escalate. If this approach doesn't work, you can bring a claim of clinical negligence against any health care provider if the care isn't of an acceptable standard and injury or death result. Care is not of an acceptable standard if it is not in accordance with what a responsible body of medical opinion would approve. Try talking to the patient advice and liaison service (PALS) or the complaints manager at the NHS trust hospital or primary care trust involved if you're worried about your care. (Ask for the details at the reception of your GP surgery or hospital.) They may be able to resolve your concerns on the spot or provide you with details of how to complain at a higher level.

Seeking a second opinion

If you're not happy with a diagnosis or want to speak to another doctor about your condition, ask your GP to arrange for a second opinion from a specialist or another GP. You don't have a legal right to a second opinion, but you should feel comfortable discussing this issue with your GP.

If your doctor refers you for a second opinion, you can't insist on seeing a particular practitioner. However, if your GP refers you to someone who you don't want to see, you can simply refuse to see that person. If your GP is unsure about a diagnosis, he or she can be found negligent if he or she then fails to refer you to a specialist and you suffer as a result.

Your right to hospital treatment

If you have back or neck pain, you may need hospital treatment in two situations: First, if your GP thinks you have a serious disease such as cancer or a major inflammatory disorder – but remember that these are quite rare and cause less than one per cent of cases of back and neck pain – and second, if your pain doesn't improve after a few weeks.

You have a set of rights with respect to hospital treatment. Remember that you need a referral from your GP for NHS hospital treatment. You can't receive NHS hospital treatment without a referral, unless you go to hospital as a medical emergency. So by and large, your GP is the hospital gatekeeper. You don't have a right to see a particular hospital doctor, although if you ask to see a specific doctor the hospital tries to meet your request. By the same token, your GP can't insist on you seeing a particular doctor. You do, however, have the right to see a doctor who works in the right specialty to deal with your back or neck pain.

Leaving hospital after treatment

You shouldn't be discharged or discharge yourself from hospital until you are completely recovered and your care needs once you're out of hospital have been assessed. You should be kept fully informed of what's going on. When you visit a doctor, being informed usually implies consent to examination and treatment, but any assessment needs to take into account your wishes. For example, if a female patient asks to be examined by a female doctor, this request must be respected. Make your wishes known before you arrive, as your doctor may not be able to comply with your wishes on the spot.

You can refuse to receive treatment. By law, a doctor can't act against your instructions, so tell your doctor about any treatment that you don't want. For example, if your practitioner offers you acupuncture but you have a horror of needles, say so! No clinician wants to give treatment that a patient isn't happy with – after all, the chances of a successful outcome are less if the patient doesn't want the treatment.

Checking Out the Alternatives

More and more people look towards complementary practitioners to treat a wide variety of health problems, including back and neck pain, as a replacement for conventional methods that haven't been successful in treating their condition or as a supplement to the conventional treatment.

Some GPs are also qualified in complementary therapies and offer them as part of their NHS treatment. Other GPs are happy to refer patients to complementary practitioners. Many, however, are not, although their number is diminishing. The complementary practitioners most commonly involved in treating back and neck pain are:

- **Acupuncturists:** Acupuncture is one of the most widely practised and researched complementary therapies. Acupuncture is a branch of traditional Chinese medicine that involves inserting fine needles at selected points on the skin to balance the body's energy (chi). Chapter 10 gets right to the point of acupuncture!
- **Chiropractors:** Chiropractic is a form of spinal manipulation. We talk more about chiropractic in Chapter 11.
- **Osteopaths:** Osteopathy is another form of spinal manipulation. We get down to the bare bones of osteopathy in Chapter 11.

Access to complementary treatment on the NHS varies depending on the primary care trust in your area. You're not automatically entitled to a referral to a complementary practitioner. Before undertaking complementary treatment, discuss your choices with your GP to ensure that the treatment's right for you. Jump to Chapter 10 for lots more about complementary therapies.

Accessing Medical Reports and Health Records

Access to your own medical records has seen major changes in recent years. As far as possible, patients are entitled to be fully informed about their medical situations. After seeing a patient, many hospital doctors now send a follow-up letter to both the patient's GP and the patient.

- ✔ You have the right to see most health records held about you.

- ✔ You're entitled to know how your records are used, who has access to them, and how you arrange to see them.

- ✔ Your GP's practice and local NHS trust hospital provide this info about your rights in the form of posters and take away leaflets.

- ✔ Your medical history should be kept confidential and shouldn't be released to anyone who isn't involved in your medical care without your consent.

Being aware of the information available to you and your right to access your medical reports should help you feel more confident in dealing with these complicated and sometimes daunting situations.

To see your medical records, you must apply in writing to the medical records department of your hospital, or the practice manager of your GP's surgery.

Getting Around the Benefits Jungle

The state benefits scene is complicated and subject to change – in fact, it can be described as a jungle. Although this sounds intimidating, benefits officials make considerable efforts to put you at your ease. For example, in a leaflet on customer information issued by the Disability and Carers Service they state that benefits workers aim to recognise you as an individual and treat you with respect. In addition, they offer an easy to use complaints procedure if, sadly, you need it.

Taking time off work: Short-term absence and benefits

Your employment contract should explain clearly your employer's policy about sick pay. Different employers have varying policies regarding sick pay. The law determines the minimum amount of sick pay that you're entitled to, known as *Statutory Sick Pay* (SSP). If your back or neck pain prevents you from going to work, you're entitled to SSP from the fourth day of your absence. You can receive up to 28 weeks of SSP a year. If your employer refuses to pay SSP, that employer must explain why. If you're off work for more than eight consecutive days, your employer can request a medical certificate from your GP or hospital doctor as proof of your illness. Your employer may accept a certificate from another health care professional, such as your osteopath or acupuncturist.

Looking at long-term absence and benefits

If you've been absent from work for a long time and you've received the maximum SSP of 28 weeks, you may decide to apply for *incapacity benefit* – the state welfare earnings replacement benefit paid to people who can't work on a long-term basis. You can find out more information about incapacity benefit through the Department for Work and Pensions (DWP) benefit enquiry telephone line on 0800-882200 or your local Job Centre Plus office. See the DWP's Web site at www.dwp.gov.uk for more information.

Dealing with disability: The personal capability assessment

To establish your entitlement to benefits, during the first 28 weeks of incapacity you're assessed against your ability to do your job. This assessment is known as the *own occupation test*.

If you're absent from work for more than 28 weeks, you may have to complete a *personal capability assessment*. A trained, approved doctor assesses your ability to carry out a range of everyday activities and determines the effects that your medical condition or disability has on your ability to carry out the tasks involved in your job. This assessment sounds daunting, but the doctor carries it out in a sensitive and customer-friendly way.

The assessing doctor can't say that you don't meet the threshold of incapacity without giving or offering you a medical examination. If the doctor decides you need a medical examination, try to keep the appointment!

Disability Rights Commission

The Disability Rights Commission (DRC) is an independent body established by Act Of Parliament to eliminate discrimination against disabled people and promote equality of opportunity. The DRC offers advice and information on the Disability Discrimination Act (DDA) and is a great place to start for advice if you're disabled or caring for someone with a disability.

The DRC does the following:

🖝 Offers advice and information to disabled people, employers, and service providers.

🖝 Supports disabled people in securing their rights under the DDA.

🖝 Helps solve problems concerning disability, often without going to court or an employment tribunal through Mediation UK (call 0117-904-6661, or see www. mediationuk.org.uk)

You can contact the DRC by calling 08457-622-633 or visiting www.drc-gb.org

If you suffer disability as a result of your back or neck pain, lots of organisations offer useful advice, including the Disability Rights Commission (which we talk about in the 'Disability Rights Commission' sidebar).

You may be entitled to benefits such as incapacity benefit (which we talk about above) or *disability benefit* (such as Disability Living Allowance) in more serious cases. If you are disabled but can still work, you may get one of the disability benefits such as DLA (which is based on personal care and mobility needs, but not the ability to work).

Getting a helping hand

You may be entitled to extra help if your back or neck pain severely affects your mobility, results in disability, or if you care for someone with such problems. Your GP or local health service can put you in touch with the relevant social services, which offer various forms of assistance, including:

🖝 Personal or practical care at home

🖝 Meals on wheels

🖝 Day care

🖝 Adaptations to the home

🖝 24-hour emergency help-alarm system

Department for Work and Pensions and Access to Work

Access to Work is a service offered by the Department of Work and Pensions. The service provides advice and practical support to disabled people and their employers to help overcome work-related obstacles resulting from a disability.

Access to Work offers the following help:

✔ Provides special aids and equipment to help a disabled person function in his or her workplace.

✔ Pays for adaptations to premises or existing equipment in the workplace.

✔ Helps with the additional costs of travel to work.

Getting Personal Advice

The topic of patients' rights and state benefits is rather complicated, and all the more so when you consider that every problem has individual features. Therefore, you may need personal advice to make the most of your particular situation. All advice given by these bodies is confidential. Here are some user-friendly organisations to help you on your way:

✔ **Citizens Advice Bureau:** Every town has a Citizens Advice Bureau (CAB). Approach your local office for advice on your situation face-to-face or over the telephone. Most CABs offer home visits and some provide e-mail advice. You can find the contact details of your local CAB on the Web site: www.citizensadvice.org.uk.

✔ **Department for Work and Pensions:** www.dwp.gov.uk. Benefits Enquiry Line: 0800-882200.

✔ **Disability Rights Commission:** www.drc-gb.org. Helpline: 08457-622- 633.

✔ **Job Centre Plus:** www.jobcentreplus.gov.uk. Telephone: 08457-622- 633.

Don't suffer in silence and struggle through on your own. Always seek expert advice – lots of people and organisations are out there ready and eager to help you.

Part II
Conventional Treatment Options

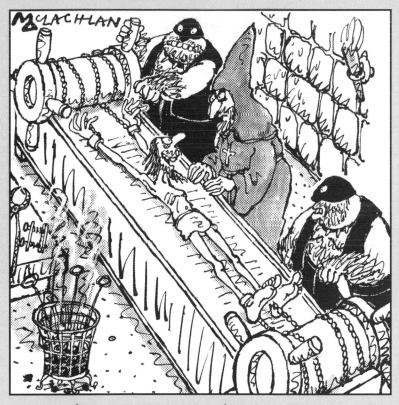

"No, no, carry on – I'm not ready
to confess yet – this is doing my
bad back no end of good."

In this part . . .

*W*hen back pain strikes, your first reaction is probably some very basic self-care, such as ice packs or heating pads, bed rest, and over-the-counter painkillers. If the pain continues for more than a couple of days, your next stop is most likely your GP, who, depending on the type and severity of pain you're experiencing, may or may not refer you to a specialist.

This part explores all these traditional treatment options. We also explain common medical tests and treatments, and we spend a chapter discussing back surgery, concentrating on whether and when it may be appropriate for you.

Chapter 6

Home Remedies: First Aid for Your Back or Neck

So things seem to be going along relatively smoothly. You have your job, you have your family and friends, and you make time to have a little fun. Then, like a bolt out the blue, your back or neck pain hits. You may have a slight pain and stiffness in your lower back or neck area. Or the pain may significantly restrict your movements and cause you distress. You may even have pain running down one or both legs.

Perhaps you've just hit the perfect drive on the eighth hole of your favourite golf course. Maybe you lifted a heavy piece of equipment at work or bent over to pick up a pencil. Or maybe you just woke up with pain one morning. In any case, the pain struck and got your attention in a major way.

Fortunately, all is not lost. Whatever your situation, you can choose from several techniques – which we discuss in this chapter – to help you manage your pain successfully.

Heading to Your GP

You can manage and treat most episodes of back or neck pain on your own. But you need to recognise the following warning signs that mean you need to forget the home remedies and go straight to your GP for an evaluation:

✔ **You can't control your bowel or bladder.** If you suddenly lose control of your bowel or bladder, see your GP or go to your local hospital accident and emergency (A&E) department *immediately*. Bowel or bladder problems include the following:

- You can't control or initiate urination or bowel movements.

- You have no feeling in your groin and/or anal area.

- You're male and you can no longer get an erection.

Any of the symptoms listed above indicate possible *cauda equina syndrome*. In the cauda equina syndrome, some of the nerves that control your bowel, bladder, and other functions become compressed. If this compression isn't corrected surgically within about 24–48 hours, these problems may become permanent due to nerve damage. (We describe cauda equina syndrome in more detail in Chapter 9.)

✔ **Your legs or feet are weak.** If you experience weakness in your legs and feet, see your GP or go to A&E within 24 hours. Weakness that occurs in your foot is called *foot drop* because you have trouble flexing your foot and toes towards your head. You may also have trouble walking because your foot is weak and has a tendency to drag.

✔ **Your back or neck pain awakens you at night.** Back or neck pain that awakens you from sleep at night can indicate a tumour or spinal infection. This type of pain – called *rest pain* – involves severe throbbing and aching that worsens with rest. Although many people with spinal pain report being awakened at night by the pain, their pain is not a constant pain that isn't altered by changes in position or getting up and walking around for a few minutes. Although a tumour or spinal infection may not be quite the emergency that the cauda equina syndrome can be (we describe this earlier in this section and in Chapter 9), you still need to see a specialist within a few days or go to A&E. While these conditions are potentially more serious than a routine attack of back or neck pain, appropriate specialist management is often very effective.

✔ **You experience significant trauma such as a car accident or a fall.** In general, when you suffer a significant trauma that causes back or neck pain, you need to see your GP or go to A&E. Your doctor may recommend an X-ray or other imaging tests to see whether you fractured any vertebrae during the trauma. If you have fractured the vertebrae, you need referring to an orthopaedic surgeon.

✔ **Your pain is excruciating.** If your back or neck pain is simply unbearable or your pain increases significantly, see your GP or go to A&E *immediately*. *Excruciating* is a subjective term, but if your pain's so bad that you can barely move or you're on the verge of tears, don't be tough – have the pain checked out.

Using Home Remedies

The following home remedies can help you manage your own back or neck pain in the initial stages or during a flare up. Keep in mind the warning symptoms we discuss in the section 'Heading to Your GP' to determine whether you need to see a doctor.

If your pain worsens as you use any of the home remedies we describe here, see your GP.

As well as the home treatments we suggest in this section, you may also consider wearing a brace, collar, or corset, applying a topical anti-inflammatory to sore muscles (ask your doctor or pharmacist to recommend a topical anti-inflammatory), having your muscles lightly massaged and stretched (check out Chapter 8 for more on massage), and engaging in deep breathing and other relaxation exercises (which we talk about in Chapters 12 and 13). Always avoid placing direct pressure on or over your spine.

Braces, collars, and corsets may be helpful but discontinue their use as soon as the pain permits. Chapter 8 has more about braces, collars, and corsets.

Climb into bed – but not for too long!

In the early stages of back or neck pain or during a significant flare up of pain, the pain may be signalling that something is wrong, such as a muscle spasm or sprain–strain.

The best course in the early stages of spinal pain is to let your pain be your guide. In other words, listen to the pain and stop what you're doing. If you're in the middle of a sporting activity, you may want to call it a day after doing some cooling-down movements such as stretching or gentle walking. If you're at work, you may want to tell your supervisor and take a break or go home for the rest of the day. Your response to the pain you're experiencing depends on the degree of the pain. For the sake of this discussion, we assume that your pain is fairly severe, requiring you to stop your activities and go home to bed.

In the old days (about ten years ago), doctors recommended weeks of strict bed rest for back or neck pain. The idea was to rest your back or neck until the pain resolved. Today, however, most practitioners believe long-term bed rest is one of the worst things you can do. Limit your overall bed rest to about two or three days – or up to five days if the pain is severe enough.

Taking extended bed rest for your back or neck pain can lead to muscle weakness, decreased flexibility, stomach and bowel problems, and ultimately an increase in your pain. Staying fairly active helps to avoid these negative aspects, even in the initial stages of your pain. For instance, in the first day or two of your back or neck pain, you may find you can only walk from your bed to the bathroom and back. Shortly thereafter, try to increase your out-of-bed time and walk more, even if you just wander around the house. Expand this activity as you feel able or as your GP guides you.

After two or three days of bed rest, aim to increase your level of activity. Try more walking or being up and out of bed for more time each day. If you have back pain, try a few gentle knee-to-chest stretches (see Chapter 15). To increase movement, you may also try other exercises – we describe lots of exercises in Chapter 15. If your pain's so severe that you don't feel that you can increase your movement after about two or three days of bed rest, consult your GP.

Resting the right way

Getting bed rest for your back or neck pain isn't as straightforward as it sounds. You should still feel free to get up occasionally to go to the bathroom and take a lap or two around your home. In fact, try to get some movement at least two to four times per day.

While resting in bed you may be tempted to prop yourself up on some pillows and watch TV or read a book. However, propping yourself up actually puts more pressure on your discs than standing and can cause more pain.

You can assume two optimal positions for your painful spine when you're in bed (see Figure 6-1):

- ✔ Lie on your side and bend at your hips and knees to 90 degrees. Place a small pillow between your knees.
- ✔ Lie on your back with your legs elevated by pillows to put your body in a position similar to the second illustration in Figure 6-1. In this position your hips and knees are bent, and the stress and pressure on your spine is at a minimum.

Sleeping on your front places your spine in a slightly extended position that can cause more pain. If you can't avoid sleeping on your front, try placing a pillow or towel under your abdomen to straighten out your spine.

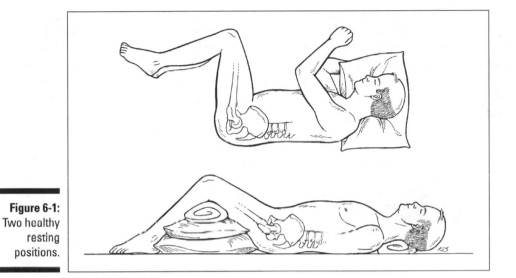

Figure 6-1:
Two healthy
resting
positions.

Getting in and out of bed

You may need a special technique to help you get in and out of the bed without significantly increasing your back pain. To get out of bed, try the following:

1. **Lie on your side, facing the side of the bed from which you plan to get out.**

   See the first illustration in Figure 6-2.

2. **Lying on your side, work your way to the edge of the bed.**

   Take care not to fall out of bed!

3. **Keeping your back straight, use your lower arm and then the palm of your hand to push yourself up slowly to a sitting position.**

   As you push yourself up, allow your legs to fall over the edge of the bed and gently to the floor. You're now in a sitting position on the bed, with your feet planted firmly on the floor. See the second illustration in Figure 6-2.

4. **From this position, you can make a smooth transition from the sitting to the standing position.**

   If you have trouble going from the sitting to the standing position, you may want to hold on to the bed head or another stable piece of furniture as you stand up.

If you feel weak or unsafe going from sitting to standing on your own, ask someone to help you, or use an *assisting device* such as a walking cane or stick – your GP can advise you on choosing an assisting device.

Try to do as much as you can for yourself, to help to work the muscles in your back and keep them strong. Getting help or using a device reduces the exercise benefit of keeping moving. You're better moving with a little help than not moving at all.

Try to do this entire movement without twisting or bending your spine. Keeping your abdominal and gluteal (buttock) muscles tight can help you perform this movement more safely.

To get into bed, simply follow steps 1–4 above in reverse. Remember to move slowly and smoothly.

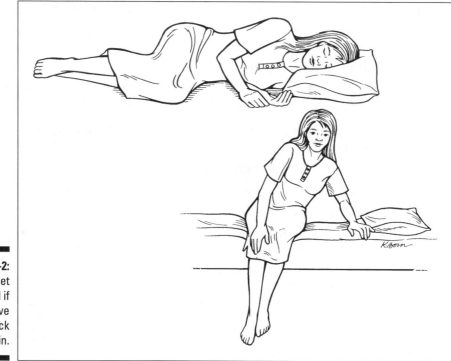

Figure 6-2:
How to get
out of bed if
you have
severe back
pain.

Cool down and heat up

Ice and heat can go a long way to relieving your back or neck pain. Here's how ice and heat work:

- ✔ Ice reduces inflammation initially by slowing down the nerves conduction, thereby providing pain relief.

- ✔ Heat causes blood vessels to expand, allowing more blood to flow to the affected area, thereby encouraging healing.

You can apply ice to your pain in a number of ways: Place ice cubes in a plastic bag and then place that in a damp tea towel on the painful area; use an ice pack, which you can buy from a pharmacy; or simply use a bag of frozen peas. (No kidding!)

Never apply ice directly to your skin, because it can freeze the skin and damage the soft tissue. You can apply the ice for up to 20 minutes every two hours.

You can also apply heat in a number of different ways: Heat a moist towel in the microwave, buy a moist heating pad from your pharmacy, or use a microwavable wheat bag.

Don't make your towel or heating pad so hot that it burns your skin or makes you uncomfortable.

One of the most common questions patients ask us is when to apply cold and when to apply heat. Take a look at two common ideas about when to apply ice and heat:

- ✔ Most doctors suggest applying ice or heat as feels best for you. This decision may include predominantly one or the other option – whichever seems to provide the most benefit for you. You can alternate ice and heat if that feels good.

- ✔ Other doctors recommend using ice in the first 48 hours after the injury and then using heat. The rationale behind this technique is that ice helps reduce inflammation and provides more pain relief. After the initial swelling decreases, heat can help healing by causing more blood flow to the area.

Both of these methods work well, and both ice and heat can reduce muscle spasm.

Try anti-inflammatory drugs

In addition to bed rest and applying ice and heat, you can use anti-inflammatory medications to help your back pain in the initial stages. Anti-inflammatories include readily available medicines such as aspirin, ibuprofen, and naproxen sodium (see Chapter 8 for more on these and other drugs). Anti-inflammatory medications decrease the inflammation associated with your back or neck pain and can provide some pain relief. However, to avoid the side effects associated with anti-inflammatories, we recommend you try paracetamol as a painkiller first.

Take all medications according to the directions on the bottle. If you think your moderate to severe back or neck pain may last for more than a day, continue taking the medicine for several doses – don't stop just because you feel a little better. Taking medication at regular intervals, according to the directions, for one or two weeks builds a level of the medication in your blood that can continue to fight inflammation and provide pain relief over the course of your acute pain flare up.

Don't think that if a little medicine is good, more must be better. Follow the directions on the medicine bottle unless your doctor suggests otherwise. Taking more medicine than is recommended can have serious side effects, such as liver and kidney damage.

Many anti-inflammatory medications that are now available over the counter were previously prescription-only drugs. As with all medication, follow the directions and read the warning labels.

The most common side effects of anti-inflammatory medications include stomach upsets, abnormal bleeding (especially with aspirin), and ulcers. If you have problems with your stomach or gastrointestinal system, check with your GP before taking any of these medicines. Generally paracetamol doesn't cause the stomach and gastrointestinal side effects of other medicines. But be aware that paracetamol can cause liver damage at higher doses (more than 4 grams per day or about eight tablets containing 500 milligrams of paracetamol each). Consult your pharmacist if you need advice.

If your back or neck pain doesn't improve after taking these medications and following our other recommendations in this chapter for one or two weeks, consult your GP. If you're on other medication for different medical problems, or have a medical problem in addition to your back or neck pain, *always* consult your physician before self-medicating, to help avoid any serious drug interactions.

Starting to Move and Returning to Normal Activity

After a few days of bed rest, gradually start to increase your activity and overall time out of bed. Walking is an excellent exercise that is safe for your back, gets your blood flowing, and stretches out your stiff muscles. Moving around also helps you feel like you're starting to return to a normal life.

Begin by walking around the house and progress to walking outside. Adjust your speed according to your pain, starting out slowly and eventually working your way up to fast walking. Make sure that you begin your walking programme on a level surface: When you're in the midst of an attack of back or neck pain, walking up and down hills can aggravate your pain.

When you have trouble following a walking programme initially, consider doing mild exercises in a swimming pool. This *hydrotherapy* (water workout) may involve simply getting into the pool and walking across the shallow end. This form of exercising is easier on your body because you're almost weightless in the water and you place minimal stress on your back. Also, the water prevents you from doing any jerky or rapid movements. We discuss hydrotherapy in more detail in Chapter 8.

When your walking's going relatively well, try adding in the exercises we discuss in Chapter 15. As you start to feel better, you can also begin to engage in more normal activities, usually starting with doing things around the house such as cooking and housework.

If you have none of the initial warning signs that we discuss at the beginning of the chapter, and you've followed the recommendations in this chapter for your acute back or neck attack but aren't experiencing significant relief or your pain isn't improving, visit your GP for an evaluation and recommendations on further treatment options.

Chapter 7

Back and Neck Pain Under the Microscope: Common Medical Tests

. . . .

In This Chapter

▶ Getting a good history and physical examination

▶ Asking questions about your testing

▶ Understanding the medical tests used for back and neck pain

. . . .

*Y*our back or neck hurts. In fact, your back or neck has been hurting for quite some time now. You may have seen your GP, a chiropractor, or a massage therapist. Or maybe you've been treating your pain on your own with limited bed rest, mild exercise, and painkillers. Regardless of the specific situation, if your initial treatment isn't working, you're going to be back at your GP's surgery ready for the next step in your treatment. But what is that next step?

If your initial treatment fails to alleviate your pain significantly, your GP may recommend some investigations or refer you to a specialist (Chapter 4 has more on the specialists involved in your treatment). Some of the tests are very simple and others are very high-tech: Not all the tests may be right for you. This chapter explains the most common tests used in back and neck pain and gives you the background you need to have an informed dialogue with your practitioner.

Appreciating the Importance of Your Medical History and Physical Examination

In recent years, we've seen an explosion in the number of high-tech approaches to assessing back and neck pain. However, even with technology on his or her side, your doctor gains the most important information by asking you about the history of your back or neck problem and by giving you a physical examination. A psychological assessment of your pain may also be an essential component in determining the correct treatment for you. (See Chapter 3 for more on how your mind influences your pain.)

Getting personal

The most important diagnostic tool with respect to your pain is a complete and thorough medical history. Your doctor should take this history in a face-to-face interview with you, in conjunction with giving you a physical examination.

To be thorough and complete, the history needs to assess *at least* the following factors:

- **How your pain started:** Did you have an accident, or did you wake up with the pain one day?

- **The course of your symptoms:** Are your symptoms getting better or worse from the time you first noticed them? Are you experiencing any new symptoms? Have any symptoms come and gone?

- **Your current symptoms:** Mention all the symptoms you currently experience, including not only your pain, but also any weakness, sleep problems, depression, and so on.

- **How the pain influences your day-to-day life:** Has your pain interrupted your work, play, family, or sexual activities in any way?

- **Whether the pain interferes with your relationships:** Are you still going out, or are you staying home more often because of the pain? Do you see people other than family members?

Assessing on the whole

After taking your medical history and physically examining you, a health care practitioner who is well trained in spinal disorders has a relatively clear idea of an appropriate treatment plan. Your practitioner conducts the physical examination to confirm his or her diagnosis based on your history. To get a good idea of your back or neck pain problem, your practitioner may assess both physical and emotional issues.

One of the primary problems we often see in the health care community is that many health care professionals focus almost entirely on physical factors to the exclusion of emotional factors. An assessment of the entire person – including both body and mind – is extremely important.

Getting physical

A thorough physical examination helps your practitioner determine whether, for example, you have a disc problem in your spine – and if so, where in your spine the problem has occurred. Your practitioner can obtain this information without using any high-tech tests.

During the physical examination, your practitioner may conduct some standard evaluations, such as taking your blood pressure and listening to your heart and lungs. He or she may assess various general attributes, such as how you walk, stand, and sit. Your practitioner may ask you to take up certain positions to see whether doing so increases your back or neck pain. He or she may push gently on areas of your body where you feel pain and use a rubber hammer to test your reflexes.

As well as these more general tests, your practitioner may do some special tests that focus more on your spine, such as the following:

✔ **Straight-leg test (sciatic nerve stretch test):** In this test, you lie flat on your back, with your legs and feet extended fully on the examination table. The practitioner lifts your legs, one at a time, to see whether doing so causes pain in either leg. This test increases the tension in the *sciatic nerve*, the nerve that goes from your back down your legs. If the test causes you pain, your practitioner can determine whether you have an irritated nerve root.

✔ **Lasegue's test:** In conjunction with a straight-leg test, your doctor may also perform Lasegue's test. In this test, you lie on your back and your practitioner brings your ankle and foot up towards your knee (one leg at a time) to put further tension on the nerves in your back that go down your legs.

To better understand the reasons for the straight-leg and Lasegue's tests, think of yourself as a puppet with nerves for strings. Your sciatic nerve is the string going from your spine to the tips of your toes. These tests pull on the string to see whether doing so causes pain. Pain during these tests indicates a problem at the *nerve root*, where the nerve leaves the spine, such as in a disc. (See Chapter 2 for more on spinal anatomy.)

✔ **Detailed evaluation of the nerves in your neck, arms, hips, legs, and feet:** Your practitioner may run a painless pinwheel device along your skin to check your sensations in these areas. The doctor looks for any changes in sensation that suggest your nerves aren't working properly. Normally you feel a slight sensation of the pinwheel running over your skin. If you feel it too much – discomfort or pain – or too little – numbness – your doctor will notice.

✔ **Reflex test:** Your doctor assesses your body's reflexes using a small rubber hammer to check that the nerves leaving your spine are working properly.

✔ **Muscular strength test:** Your practitioner may assess the strength of the muscle groups in your body. Each of these muscle groups corresponds to a specific *nerve-root level*, the part of your lower spine where the nerve exits the spine. If a nerve is injured, the muscles it controls may be weak.

If your doctor focuses only on finding a problem in your spine, the diagnosis and treatment may be incomplete or even incorrect. Your practitioner needs to assess your pain from a viewpoint of you as a whole person – mind, body, personal history, and so on.

After taking your medical history and physically examining you, your practitioner may recommend a treatment plan or further diagnostic testing.

A detailed and appropriate history and physical examination are more critical than ever. Without these, your doctor can't look at a high-tech study and properly identify clinically significant changes.

Examining Your Doctor

Ideally, you need to feel that you and your doctor are partners in your treatment. You have the right to ask your doctor questions about your treatment and diagnostic testing. Be sure to exercise this right: If your practitioner isn't interested in answering your questions, you may want to consider seeing another doctor by asking for a referral. See Chapter 24 for more about working in partnership with your doctor.

Try asking your doctor the following questions if he recommends you have any diagnostic tests:

- **What makes up the test and what does it show?** Ask for the proper name of the test and what your doctor hopes to find out. For example, your doctor may reply: 'I'm recommending an MRI, which shows all the tissues of your spine, including the discs, bones, and nerves.'

- **Why do you advise I have this test?** Find out what information your doctor expects to get from this test.

- **What can I expect before, during, and after the test?** Try to get some idea of what the test involves. How long is it going to take? Do you have to prepare beforehand in any way? Is the test uncomfortable or painful?

- **How will the results change my treatment or prognosis?** This question homes in on how your doctor expects to use the test results and what those results mean for your treatment.

If your practitioner doesn't consider all aspects of you – physical, psychological, and emotional – the results of your diagnostic tests are of little value and can even be detrimental to you if you experience side effects to no purpose.

Exploring Your Diagnostic Testing Options

In this section, we describe several diagnostic tests that your practitioner may suggest to investigate your back or neck pain. Although the interpretation of the tests may be complicated, you can still understand what the test involves, what it shows, why having it makes sense for you, and what side effects it may have.

Keep in mind that your practitioner needs to assess you as an entire person – mind and body – and not just as a spine that happens to come with a human being wrapped around it. The results of these tests (except the psychological tests) are meaningless if they're not combined with your medical history and physical examination. Although many diagnostic tests are high-tech and sound impressive, they often don't identify the cause of your back or neck pain. Even without a diagnosis, you can still treat and manage your back or neck pain to a certain extent.

Plain X-Rays

An X-ray machine passes low-level radiation through the part of your body being examined, projecting a picture, or *radiograph*, on to a piece of film. The level of radiation from an X-ray is very small.

Your doctor may recommend you have an X-ray to show the bones of your spine, sacroiliac joint, and pelvis. An X-ray can show whether you're experiencing changes associated with normal ageing, fractures, and the overall alignment of your spine. (For more about spinal alignment problems, such as scoliosis, see Chapter 3.) You may be an appropriate candidate for an X-ray when:

✔ You still have pain after two or three weeks of conservative treatment.

✔ You have pain even during periods of no activity.

✔ You have pain that awakens you from sleep at night.

✔ You have pain after a trauma or fall.

Generally, your doctor shouldn't recommend an X-ray on your first visit unless, for example, he or she suspects a fracture due to trauma, or if you've had pain for a long time before seeing your doctor. When your back or neck pain begins after an accident such as a fall or a car accident, you can reasonably expect to have an X-ray. In all other cases, your doctor needs to take a full history and physical examination to determine whether an X-ray is necessary.

Having an X-ray is simple and painless. The person performing the test may cover sensitive areas of your body (such as genitalia) with a lead shield. X-rays aren't safe for women during pregnancy, but otherwise they aren't harmful and have no side effects provided that these precautions are taken.

Supposedly 'abnormal' findings on your X-ray, such as wear-and-tear changes that occur with ageing (given the scary name 'degenerative changes'), usually aren't significant and often don't relate to your pain. Findings that may relate to your spinal pain include such conditions as fractures, severe degeneration, and significant scoliosis (which we describe in Chapter 3).

Just because your X-rays don't show anything significant doesn't mean that your pain isn't real. The majority of painful spinal conditions arise from the soft tissues of your spine, including the muscles, tendons, discs, and ligaments: Unfortunately, X-rays see right through these so if you do have problems in these tissues they won't show up on X-ray.

MRI (magnetic resonance imaging)

Magnetic resonance imaging (MRI) uses a strong magnetic field, radio waves, and a computer to generate a picture of your spinal structures.

An MRI shows the nerves, muscles, ligaments, discs, and bones of your spine. This test gives your doctor much more information than an X-ray without exposing you to any radiation.

An MRI may be appropriate for you when:

✔ You are considering having surgery for your pain. (We cover spinal surgery in Chapter 9.)

✔ Your doctor suspects your pain may be related to an infection or tumour. (Severe pain that awakens you from sleep is often a symptom of an infection or tumour.)

Because the MRI test is extremely sensitive, your doctor can detect subtle changes in your spine that occur naturally as you age. However, the good news is that these changes occur in people without back pain, so you can be fairly confident that these changes aren't causing your pain – especially when you are older than 35.

MRI is generally safe. However, pregnant women may be at some risk of premature labour. If you're pregnant, work with your doctor to determine the best course of testing for you.

The MRI procedure is safe, has almost no side effects, and requires no special preparation. You lie down on a scanning table that slides into a giant magnetic tube. If you're claustrophobic, the closeness of the tube may make you a little uncomfortable. Ask your doctor in advance to arrange for you to receive a sedative. You may also be given special glasses to wear to protect your eyes, and headphones through which to listen to music to lessen your anxiety – some scanning units allow you to bring your own music. Some hospitals, although not many, have open scanners (perfect if you have claustrophobia).

Inside the tube, you hear several noises, including a humming sound and a thumping as the radio waves are turned on and off. Generally, the most difficult part of the test is lying still for 45–60 minutes, especially if your back or neck hurts at the time. If your pain is severe, you may consider asking your doctor for some pain relief before the test.

Some MRI tests involve injecting a contrast agent into your arm or leg before the test. A *contrast agent* is a non-harmful substance that makes the MRI picture much clearer, especially if you've had spine surgery. The contrast agent helps your doctor distinguish scar tissue, which may occur following surgery.

An MRI can't show certain causes of pain, such as a sprain or strain in the muscles or ligaments and stress-related pain. Therefore, you can have normal test results and still have pain.

CT (computerised tomography) scanning

A CT scan is a computerised recording of a slice or section of your body. You may know the test by the name *CAT scan – computerised axial tomography*.

CT scanning exposes you to a greater amount of radiation than a plain X-ray, but the amount is still well within the safe range. The CT scan doesn't show your soft tissues, nerves, and muscles quite as well as MRI, but does show the anatomy of the bony structures of your spine, your discs, and nerves.

Your doctor may suggest CT scanning rather than MRI when:

- You're very claustrophobic and can't tolerate being in the MRI machine even with a sedative.
- Your doctor needs to see the anatomy of your bony structures where the nerves leave your spinal canal.

The CT scanner is a cylinder-shaped machine, just like the MRI machine. You lie on your back for about 30–45 minutes. The tube portion of the CT scanner is much larger than the MRI tube and less likely to make you feel claustrophobic.

The CT scan is painless. As with MRI, your doctor may recommend you have the scan with a contrast agent to make the scan clearer.

Myelography

A *myelogram* is an X-ray of the fluid-filled sac around your spinal cord. In myelography, the radiologist injects an amount of dye into this sac, which helps the area show up on the X-ray. A *radiologist* is a doctor who specialises in imaging tests, such as X-rays, MRI, and CT scanning.

Sometimes you have a CT scan immediately after a myelogram. By combining the two tests, your doctor can see your bones or skeletal structure and neuro-logical structures, such as the nerves, and you need have only one injection.

Generally, myelography is appropriate only when you and your doctor are considering surgery, your MRI or CT scan image isn't clear, your doctor can't make a specific diagnosis from the scan, or your doctor suspects you have a tumour.

Myelography may cause minimal to moderate pain in the form of a headache following the procedure. Because of new technology and improved safety, this test no longer requires a hospital stay and is now often done on an out-patient basis. You lie on a table as the radiologist injects dye into your spinal canal – a process that takes one or two minutes. You may feel a slight prick-ing sensation as the radiologist inserts the needle. After the dye is injected, the technician takes X-rays of you in many positions, including standing, par-tially upright, lying down, and turned to the right or left side. A CT scan may follow. The entire process takes about an hour.

After the test, the recovery period is about 6–12 hours. In the hospital, you may be asked to lie down with your head slightly elevated and to drink plenty of fluids. Following these recommendations keeps the contrast material away from sensitive areas in your head and flushes the material out of your body.

You may experience a headache after myelography for one of two reasons:

- ✔ **You may react to the dye:** Less than 1 per cent of people who undergo myelography have a reaction to the dye. The good news is that over the past five years, newer, water-soluble dyes have become available, which have fewer side effects.

- ✔ **A small amount of spinal fluid may leak out into your body through the needle hole:** This occurs in 5–10 per cent of people undergoing myelography. The resulting headache lasts for one to two days following the test. The headache almost always subsides when you rest for a few hours and drink plenty of fluids. Otherwise the headache may take a few days to subside.

Myelography is a very low risk procedure, although it carries slightly more risk than X-rays, MRIs, and CT scans. Myelography has two very rare risks, which are infection and excessive bleeding. If you get an infection following myelography, your doctor can treat it with antibiotics, and excessive bleed-ing may be treated with a blood transfusion.

To prevent excessive bleeding as a result of clotting problems, don't take aspirin or any blood thinning medication for three to five days before your myelography test.

Bone scanning

In a *bone scan*, you have an injection in the arm with a special radioactive dye. The radioactivity involved is extremely low-level and safe. You lie down for about two hours while the dye circulates throughout your entire body, including your bones.

After the dye has circulated throughout your body, you have special X-rays taken to determine how much of the dye has penetrated into various parts of your skeleton. The scan works by detecting any parts of your skeleton that have an increase in blood flow due to more activity in the cells. The increase in blood flow can result from a tumour, infection, fracture, or age-related degenerative changes. Your doctor may recommend a bone scan when he or she can't diagnose any of these conditions by plain X-rays, MRI, or CT scanning.

Bone scanning is very safe. The test is generally risk-free, although if you have moderate to severe back pain you may have difficulty lying down for such a long time as you wait for the dye to circulate.

The most common mistake made in interpreting bone scans is to attribute too much significance to findings that result from arthritic or normal wear-and-tear changes in the bones of the spine. See Chapter 2 for more details on anatomy.

Discography

In discography, dye is injected directly into the discs of your lumbar spine. The dye helps create a better picture of this area of your spine, and the doctor can determine whether injecting the dye in a specific disc causes the type of pain that you have been experiencing. You may experience moderate to severe pain during this test. Of all the tests we discuss in this chapter, most patients say that this is the most uncomfortable. However, discography has few side effects, apart from infection very rarely.

Your practitioner may recommend a discography test when your MRI shows disc bulges or herniations at more than one spinal level (see Chapter 3 for more on bulges and herniations). The discogram helps identify which, if any, of the disc herniations or bulges are responsible for your pain. A discogram may also help determine whether a degenerative disc is the source of your back or neck pain.

Only agree to discography if you're willing to consider surgical treatment based on the test results, otherwise you'll have undergone an unpleasant experience for no purpose.

Electrodiagnostic studies

Electromyography (EMG) and nerve conduction studies (NCS) are the most common *electrodiagnostic studies* – tests that measure the electrical activity and function of your nerves and muscles to assess your pain. The tests show whether the electrical activity of various nerves has been disrupted.

A rheumatologist or neurologist usually does these tests, so you may be referred to another doctor if your practitioner doesn't specialise in this type of testing.

During the study, the practitioner inserts small needles into several of the muscles to be measured. In an EMG, these needles are connected to a monitor showing the electrical activity of your nerves and muscles. In an NCS, an electrical pulse 'buzzes' your nerves and special electrodes monitor the electrical activity in those nerves. You may experience mild to moderate pain with both EMG and NCS tests.

Electrodiagnostic studies can help determine a variety of diagnoses involving the nervous system and assess the regrowth of nerves after you've had lumbar-disc surgery for sciatica. Your doctor can make most diagnoses following a good history and physical examination and some of the other diagnostic tests mentioned in this chapter, and so electrodiagnostic studies are becoming less necessary.

Moving from Body to Mind

Some people are surprised to find that psychological testing often goes hand-in-hand with the other diagnostic tests we discuss in this chapter. A number of psychological tests have been designed or adapted for use with people with back or neck pain. Your doctor may recommend these tests as part of a pre-surgical screening, to assess the emotional aspects of your pain or ongoing psychiatric problems, or to assess your ability to cope with the pain.

Just as the history and physical examination are the most important parts of diagnosing your back or neck pain problem, the clinical interview is the key psychological assessment tool.

Your doctor may suggest a psychological assessment of your back or neck pain if he or she thinks that

  ✔ You may have significant depression and/or anxiety.

  ✔ You may be abusing alcohol or other substances, or overusing pain medicines.

  ✔ You're unable to cope with the pain.

  ✔ You're experiencing undue stress in your family or work situation.

  ✔ You may benefit from psychological pain-control procedures.

  ✔ You may benefit from psychological preparation for surgery.

  ✔ Your pain may be stress-related.

A psychologist or psychiatrist with special training in pain problems usually conducts the psychological assessment. In the interview, the practitioner asks you for information about the history of your pain problem, including previous treatments, your family and work situations, litigation/compensation issues related to your pain, your history of previous psychological treatment, any substance abuse problems, and your history of emotional and/or physical abuse. In addition, the practitioner may conduct special examinations to assess your mood, sleep, memory, concentration abilities, changes in your sex life, and energy levels.

Psychological testing reveals information about many aspects of your pain, including:

- ✔ Your level of depression and anxiety related to your pain
- ✔ Your personality features and how they affect your experience of pain
- ✔ Whether you're comfortable in the sick role
- ✔ Whether you're more dramatic or stoic in showing pain behaviours
- ✔ Whether non-physical factors (emotions, family, work, and so on) are likely to be influencing your pain

You may find a referral for psychological assessment threatening. For instance, you may feel that your doctor is 'dumping' you or thinks your pain is 'in your head', not your spine. In truth, the purpose of the evaluation is to help your doctor determine the best treatment approach for you. The evaluation can also determine which, if any, psychological pain-control methods may help you, such as relaxation training (which we talk about in Chapter 13), changing the way you view your pain, and helping your family members cope with your pain.

All pain is real and includes emotional or psychological factors. If your practitioner refers you for a psychological assessment, don't think that you're starring in a re-enactment of *One Flew Over the Cuckoo's Nest*! If your doctor states or implies that your pain is imaginary, consider finding another health care professional.

Chapter 8

Going the Conservative Treatment Route

. . . .

. . . .

*W*hen you hear the word 'conservative', you may immediately think of politics and economics. In the world of spinal pain, though, 'conservative' applies to any treatment that doesn't involve surgery. Most common medical treatments are conservative.

Conservative treatments fall into two categories: invasive and non-invasive. Non-invasive techniques are further broken down into active (you administer the treatment yourself) and passive (someone else gives you the treatment – usually a physiotherapist). Most treatments for spinal pain are non-invasive and include treatments such as physiotherapy and medication. Invasive approaches include mad-scientist-sounding measures such as trigger point injections, nerve blocks, and 'implantable' pain therapies. This chapter introduces the non-invasive and invasive conservative approaches available to you.

Although some of the invasive treatments can sound frightening, keep in mind that they're all non-surgical treatments. And remember that nothing substitutes for an open dialogue with your practitioner. Sharing your thoughts gives your practitioner the opportunity to alleviate your fears, address your concerns, and explore other treatment options.

The doctor dialogue

Having an active partnership with your doctor or other health care practitioner is one of the most important aspects of any treatment you receive for your back or neck pain. As part of this active participation, you need to make sure that you understand thoroughly why your practitioner recommends a particular treatment and what you can expect from it. Try asking the following questions:

✔ Why are you recommending this treatment for me?

✔ What benefit can I expect, and how long before I know whether that benefit has been achieved?

✔ What problems may occur with this treatment? If these problems do occur, what do I do? Are these problems likely to go away if I continue with the treatment?

✔ Is this treatment going to interfere with other treatments I'm pursuing? (You may want to give a list of the names and phone numbers of everyone involved in your treatment to all your practitioners.)

Analysing Active Therapies

Active treatments include general exercise, exercise programmes, and special back and neck exercises. You actively do these treatments for yourself, under the guidance of a professional.

Exercising healthily

Exercise is one of the most important treatments to help your pain. Your practitioner may refer you to a physiotherapist who is an expert in exercise treatments. Your physiotherapist may suggest an exercise programme, with exercises that strengthen specific areas of your back and neck. An exercise programme has the goals of increasing your strength, improving your flexibility, improving the way you move, and building your endurance. Specialised exercise programmes have fancy names such as *flexion*, *extension*, and *lumbar stabilisation* (we talk about these in Chapter 15).

Conditioning your body

Conditioning exercises, which focus more on total body fitness than on specific pain, need to be the key component of your rehabilitation programme. This type of programme incorporates activities such as cycling on a stationary bike, using a treadmill, and following a walking programme.

An exercise programme can help you:

- ✔ **Manage your fear of back or neck pain:** Exercise requires you to move around. As well as exercising your body, including your spine, exercise reassures you that you don't have to fear your pain or protect your body's movements.

- ✔ **Change the 'hurt equals harm' mindset:** A proper exercise programme helps you accept that increased pain doesn't necessarily mean injury. Your pain may initially increase when you start to exercise, but in reality, this type of pain is often the same as anyone experiences after not exercising for a while.

- ✔ **Escape the sick role:** An exercise programme also helps you address any issues that may be forcing you to maintain the *sick role*. When you exercise and move around, other people don't think of you as a sick person. As they begin to treat you as a healthy person, your attitude and confidence may well improve.

An exercise programme can be appropriate whatever the stage of your back or neck pain. Generally, your physiotherapist prescribes a programme tailored to your specific back or neck pain.

Your practitioner should evaluate you carefully before prescribing an exercise programme to ensure that you have no physical problems, such as spinal instability or a fractured vertebra (see Chapter 3), that can make exercise harmful. Medical problems such as heart disease and high blood pressure can also change the type of programme your practitioner recommends. Don't forget to tell your practitioner if you're on any medication or if you're pregnant.

The pedometer: a simple but powerful tool

A pedometer is a small device attached to your belt that 'counts' the number of steps you take. Walkers and joggers often wear electronic pedometers to measure the number of steps they take and the distance they travel. Pedometers are inexpensive and can help you keep track of your overall activity level as you try to overcome your back or neck pain.

Several researchers have found that using a pedometer provides an accurate assessment of the degree to which you're engaging in normal levels of healthy activity. For example, some experts advise that healthy people aim for levels of 10,000 steps a day. In contrast, a study of people with rheumatoid arthritis showed an average of 5,037 steps a day. A good way to use a pedometer is to gather baseline information over a few days to measure your usual level of activity. You can then compare your increase in activity relative to your baseline. For more about using your baseline activity to further develop your strength and stamina, see the sidebar 'Using the quota system' in this chapter.

Taking responsibility

Ultimately, you're responsible for your own health. Bear in mind the following points as you start an exercise programme:

✔ **Your pain may increase initially:** When you begin an exercise programme, you may use muscles you've 'protected' for quite a while. As a result, you may experience a mild to moderate increase in pain. This pain does *not* mean that you're injuring your back or neck, and the initial pain is likely to decrease over time.

✔ **You need to follow the programme independently:** Your practitioner or physiotherapist may monitor you closely at the beginning of the programme and then instruct you to go ahead and complete the exercises on your own. To really conquer your pain, you need to follow through with the programme on your own.

✔ **You must comply with the exercise recommendations:** Cutting short the exercises can be very tempting, especially when your physiotherapist isn't monitoring you – rather like cheating in class when your teacher isn't looking. Remember though: You're only cheating yourself when you take these shortcuts.

Changing your exercise programme according to your pain

Back and neck pain have different phases. Your exercise programme depends on which phase you're experiencing. With chronic back or neck pain, for instance, your muscles may be weak from inactivity. In this case, your exercise programme starts out quite slowly and builds in intensity over time. (We discuss the specifics of designing an exercise programme in the sidebar 'Using the quota system'.)

The following list shows how your physiotherapist may design your exercise programme based upon your back or neck pain phase:

✔ **Initial phase of acute pain (duration of one to five days):** Your pain and muscle spasm may be quite limiting during this phase. Your practitioner may recommend ice, bed rest, and some gentle knee-to-chest stretches on day two or three, as shown in Chapter 15.

✔ **Acute pain (duration of less than one month):** Mild exercise that you gradually increase can help you avoid the subacute stage of pain altogether. Even in this early stage of pain, mild exercise, such as limited walking, is appropriate. Over the next few weeks, you can slowly add more strenuous activities such as faster walking, swimming, or bicycling. The type of exercise you choose usually isn't important, but discuss your choice with your physiotherapist. At this stage of treatment, avoid any severe twisting or bending motions. Exercise until you experience more pain and then stop.

✔ **Subacute pain (duration of one to three months):** Exercise becomes very important in this phase. Your practitioner is trying to keep you as active as possible, even if you have ongoing pain. The exercises your practitioner gives you may increase your pain initially, but if you do the exercises as prescribed, they're designed to be safe for your spine. At this point, your doctor may monitor your physiotherapy programme more closely.

✔ **Chronic pain (duration of more than three months):** At this stage, a physical reconditioning programme including strengthening, stretching, and aerobic exercises needs to be part of your total treatment plan. As you begin to use the weakened muscles, your pain initially increases. Using some of the passive therapies we discuss later in this chapter may help control your symptoms so that you can complete your exercise programme more effectively. At this phase of exercising, your pain is no longer your guide. Instead, take a drill-sergeant approach: Work slowly through the pain by completing a certain number of repetitions of each exercise, regardless of the pain.

✔ **Recurrent acute pain (pain flare ups punctuated by pain-free episodes):** Participating in an aerobic exercise programme about three times a week can significantly decrease the frequency, intensity, and duration of your back or neck pain episodes. You can choose any type of exercise as long as it includes aerobic, stretching, and strengthening elements. You may want to include some specific exercises that your practitioner recommended previously.

Conditioning your back and neck

Plan your back and neck exercise programme in conjunction with your doctor and physiotherapist, and also take into account the information contained in this chapter and Chapter 15. In this section, we look at the important elements of an exercise programme. These features help you follow your exercise programme on a regular basis.

One element of your exercise programme needs to be aerobic conditioning. The aerobic conditioning components may be in addition to special exercises such as those reviewed in Chapter 15. Aerobic exercise can be anything from speed walking, to cycling on a stationary bicycle, to step-aerobics. Although aerobic conditioning isn't targeted directly to your spine, we find that this type of exercise not only helps you manage your pain more effectively but also improves your mental abilities, provides stress relief, and helps you sleep better.

Pacing your activities

Pacing means increasing your activity gradually according to a specific plan, applicable from day one. This concept involves breaking an activity up into small pieces, with breaks in between, to help prevent flare ups in your pain.

Using the quota system

The *quota system* is a special approach to your exercise programme. You work to a specific quota rather than being guided by your pain. Exercising in this way is especially important when you're in the subacute or chronic stages of back or neck pain.

To set up a quota system for any exercise, begin by establishing your *baseline.* Your baseline for that exercise is the amount of exercise you can do until pain or fatigue stops you. Your amount of exercise can be measured in several ways depending upon the type of exercise, for example the time the exercise takes, the number of repetitions, or the distance.

Record this figure for three consecutive exercise sessions to get a good measure of your baseline capabilities. Say, for example, that you can do your treadmill exercise for five minutes on the first session, six minutes on the second session, and seven minutes on the third session. In each of these sessions, stop when the pain or fatigue becomes uncomfortable.

In this example, you take the average of the three sessions to establish your baseline of six

minutes (5 + 6 + 7 = 18, divide by 3 to get 6). After you establish the baseline, subtract 20 per cent. The remaining number sets your *initial quota*. In this example, 6 – 20 per cent = 4.8. Your initial quota, therefore, is approximately five minutes.

After you establish your initial quota, complete that goal regardless of your pain. You then set increasing quotas for yourself based on discussions with your practitioner. For example, you may choose to increase your quota by 10 per cent each week or every third exercise session.

You can use the quota system for any of your exercises or activities: Try the distance you can walk, the laps you can swim, the amount of time you can sit at a desk, or your time on the treadmill. The important point to remember about quotas is that the goal is to *work to the quota* rather than to the pain. Therefore, don't make your quotas too difficult or potentially unachievable. If you can't achieve a particular quota, back off a little for a couple of sessions and then return to your previous quota goals.

Pacing your activities prevents the common pattern of *overdoing* and *crashing.* You may experience the overdo-and-crash pattern when you have minimal back pain and engage vigorously in an activity, only for the exercise to cause a flare up that sets you back. The overdo-and-crash pattern is an unhealthy approach to your pain and you need to replace the pattern with a pacing approach. *Pacing* involves doing a reasonable amount of exercise or activity, with breaks in between, so you keep your pain under reasonable control.

Don't confuse pacing yourself with letting pain be your guide. If you pace your activities, you're likely to notice that you can do more rather than less and you're less likely to experience the overdo-and-crash pattern.

Getting your family and friends involved

One of the best ways to implement your exercise programme is to get your family and friends involved. However, your family and friends may be inclined to tell you to take it easy and not be so active, even if your practitioner has told you to exercise more. In this situation, your family and friends are inadvertently keeping you in a sick role.

Explain to your family and friends about the importance of your conditioning exercise programme. Tell them about pacing and ask them to encourage you to maintain a regular, healthy regimen and to warn you if they think that you're entering overdo-and-crash mode.

Include your family and friends in your efforts to become more active by doing the following:

- **Make a public commitment:** Tell as many people as possible about your plan to increase your activities and your exercise programme to help ensure that you follow through with your programme.

- **Get an exercise buddy:** Setting up a regular exercise programme with a friend makes you less likely to cancel or drop your exercise programme.

Understanding pain and functional restoration programmes

Your practitioner may suggest that you try a pain programme if the usual treatments, such as physiotherapy, exercise, and medicines, aren't helping and your pain is quite debilitating (for instance, such that you can't work). These programmes are more common than they used to be but are still not common enough. In the vast majority of cases pain programmes are hospital-based. Your back or neck specialist (which we talk about in Chapter 1) may refer you to a pain programme.

The terms *pain programme* and *functional restoration* describe treatment programmes that have slightly different focuses. The two programmes, however, do share a few characteristics:

- **Multidisciplinary approach:** A number of different specialists work with you at the same time.

- **Structured approach:** You receive various treatments at a specific time for a specific reason.

- **Common goals:** Each programme works to decrease your pain, increase your function, and improve your quality of life.

- **Motivation driven:** Each programme relies on a high level of motivation and involvement from you.

A *functional restoration programme* focuses on helping you to eliminate any disability that your pain causes and increasing your physical and mental abilities to restore your function. The aim of these programmes is to increase your ability to participate in day-to-day activities. The treatments are primarily exercise-oriented, with a 'hurt doesn't equal harm' attitude. Instead of trying to 'fix' your pain (by the time you get to one of these programmes, the fix-it approaches may have failed), these programmes focus on what you can do to help you work through your pain safely and gradually.

Most pain programmes have a screening evaluation that looks at the type of pain you have (these programmes often treat chronic back and neck pain syndromes and failed back surgery syndrome, which we talk about in Chapter 3). These programmes have been found to be highly successful if you're a good candidate and pass the screening evaluation.

Perusing Passive Therapies

Passive treatment is something that a physiotherapist or other professional does to you. In these treatments, you're essentially a passive recipient of the treatment. This section looks at the most common passive physiotherapy treatments.

Hot and cold packs

The use of *hot and cold packs* (or some other method of alternating heat and cold) is one of the most common techniques to treat back and neck pain. The overall action of hot and cold packs (other than the obvious temperature difference) is similar. Hot packs help relax your muscles, increase local blood flow, and relieve your pain. Cold packs also help relieve your back or neck pain and decrease muscle spasm. After causing an initial decrease in blood flow, cold packs eventually cause an increase in blood flow to the affected area.

Generally, applying hot and cold packs to your back or neck provides only temporary relief. No evidence shows that hot or cold application results in any long-term benefits; however, using hot and cold packs to manage your pain can enable you to complete appropriate exercises more effectively (we describe back exercises in Chapter 15).

Ultrasound

Ultrasound waves are high frequency sound waves. Various tissues in your body absorb ultrasound waves, even though the frequency is too high for the human ear to hear. (A pity you can't say the same about some forms of music!) This absorption produces heat deep at the tissue site, below the surface of your skin. Heating the tissues in your back or neck area helps relieve your pain, increase blood flow, and promote muscle relaxation – just like hot packs.

Physiotherapists often use a combination of hot packs, cold packs, and ultrasound to help relieve your pain. The relief you feel is usually temporary, and the therapies have no long-term benefits by themselves. We recommend that you use ultrasound treatment in conjunction with an appropriate exercise programme.

Ultrasound requires special equipment and training, so a trained technician must administer the treatment. To keep you from becoming dependent on your practitioner for pain relief, we recommend that you seek these treatments only on a short-term basis (the first few weeks of your back or neck pain treatment, for instance). After that time, try to apply hot and cold packs yourself on an as-needed basis to help manage your pain as you increase your exercises.

Massage

Massage is thought to increase the blood flow to the massaged area and to relax your muscles, causing a decrease in spasm and pain. Many people tell us that massage is helpful for their pain, and you may find similar results – at least on a temporary basis. As an added bonus, massage feels great! Any massage treatment you undergo, however, needs to be part of an overall treatment plan that involves an active, appropriate exercise programme. We don't recommend massage as a treatment by itself.

Depending on the intensity of the massage approach, your pain may increase during the massage. Usually, though, muscle relaxation and pain relief quickly follow. Applying heat before massage or deep-tissue work helps loosen up your muscles. After a massage or deep-tissue work, applying ice can help relieve pain.

As with other passive physical approaches, don't become dependent solely on massage as a way to manage your back or neck pain in the long-term. Massage can be expensive and doesn't address your underlying problem.

Bed rest

Bed rest may sound great to you, because at the very least it doesn't increase your pain. However, we believe that too much bed rest and limited activity put you at risk for developing *physical deconditioning syndrome*, in which your muscles weaken, contributing to and prolonging your pain problem. (See Chapter 3 for more on physical deconditioning syndrome.)

Generally, limit your bed rest to about two to five days after the onset of severe back or neck pain and then begin to increase your activities gradually. Let your practitioner guide you into gradually resuming your activities.

Water therapy

Water's physical properties make it a good source of treatment for spinal pain. In water, you're buoyant and essentially weightless, which takes the pressure of gravity off your body, specifically your lower back area. Water also provides resistance to your movements, forcing your movement to be slow, rhythmic, and smooth. Exercises done in water often produce less pain and tend not to cause pain flare ups.

Water therapy – or *hydrotherapy* – can be active or passive. In active therapy, you actually exercise in the pool. Starting in the pool can be an excellent way to begin an exercise programme, especially if you're unfit or afraid to exercise. After a few weeks in the pool, you can graduate to a land programme.

In passive therapy, you simply sit in a jacuzzi. Treatment using a jacuzzi is essentially a passive physical therapy treatment, and we recommend that you limit your use of a jacuzzi, although this treatment may help manage your symptoms while you engage in a more active therapy.

Transcutaneous electrical nerve stimulation (TENS)

Transcutaneous electrical nerve stimulation (TENS) involves applying a mild level of electrical stimulation to the painful area of your back or neck. You place bandage-like electrodes on your skin. Wires attach the electrodes to a small battery-operated unit that passes low-level electricity between the electrodes. When the unit is switched on, you may feel a tingling going between the electrodes. A variety of TENS units are on the market, which emit electrical patterns of differing amplitude, frequencies, and pulse widths. Ask your doctor or physiotherapist about the differences.

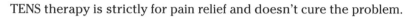

The theory behind TENS is that the mild electrical stimulation (a mild tingling sensation) overrides the pain signal coming from your spine. As the TENS unit blocks the pain signal, you begin to feel a decrease in pain.

TENS therapy is strictly for pain relief and doesn't cure the problem.

The only way to determine whether a TENS unit works for your pain is to try it. We recommend that you try TENS initially at your doctor's surgery or physiotherapy department. You may even be able to borrow a TENS unit to test it out. If you notice some pain relief with TENS, consider renting a unit for a month or so first, before purchasing one.

As with other treatments that focus on pain relief, we recommend that you use a TENS unit in conjunction with an exercise programme and increased activities.

Traction

Traction (used mainly in lower back pain) is an apparatus or manual treatment that applies *tension of distraction* to your spine in order to pull the vertebrae away from each other. Separating the vertebrae of your spine slightly is thought to relieve some of the pressure on your discs and joints. In pelvic traction, an apparatus wrapped around your hips applies distraction tension to your lower spine.

Like other passive treatments, traction can provide only temporary pain relief. Most research indicates that traction has no long-term benefits. Home traction units are available for neck pain that some people find very helpful.

Corsets, braces, and collars

At some time during your treatment, your doctor may suggest you try a corset, brace, or collar for your back or neck pain. A brace or corset can restrict motion, provide abdominal support, and correct your posture. Some conditions – such as recovering from spinal fusion surgery and fractured vertebrae – require you to wear a brace for a short period of time.

In most cases of back or neck pain, wearing a brace, corset, or collar provides temporary pain relief, especially during increased activity or while sitting for long periods of time. We recommend that you use a brace, corset, or collar in conjunction with an ongoing exercise programme as prescribed by your doctor.

Wearing a brace, corset, or collar is only a temporary measure.

Mulling Over Medications

Medication and back and neck pain don't necessarily go hand-in-hand. In conjunction with an overall treatment plan that includes such remedies as appropriate exercise, medication can help decrease your pain, reduce inflammation, and relieve muscle spasm. However, you and your doctor must decide together whether medication is a good option for you.

Whenever you take medication, try to be an informed consumer. Be aware of any potential side effects of the medication you take and whether the drug may interact with other drugs. To make sure that your treatment with medication succeeds, ask your doctor the following questions about your medication:

- ✔ Why are you recommending this medication?

- ✔ What benefit can I expect, and how long before I know whether the medication is achieving the goal?

- ✔ How do I take this medication? (Morning or night, with meals, on an empty stomach, every four hours, and so on.)

- ✔ What side effects need I be aware of? What do I do if these effects occur? Are these side effects likely to go away if I decide to stay on the medication?

- ✔ Can I take this medication in addition to the other medication I'm already on? (Make a habit of giving all your practitioners a list of your current medications for their records.)

- ✔ How do I stop taking this medication safely?

Always check that the medication you get from the pharmacy is the same one that you and your doctor discuss.

The following sections explain the various types of medication that your doctor may prescribe to treat your back or neck pain. These guidelines are general, so ensure that you're always clear about what your doctor is recommending for your unique problem. Follow your doctor's directions for taking the medication carefully.

The following categories of medication are listed in order of the most commonly used to the least commonly used. Therefore, you may expect your doctor to start with medication at the beginning of the list and move towards the end of the list if necessary. The categories are not entirely distinct and several overlap; for example, anti-inflammatory drugs also have analgesic properties.

Analgesics

Doctors commonly prescribe *analgesics* – painkillers – for back and neck pain. Analgesics vary from over-the-counter preparations, such as aspirin and paracetamol, to very strong narcotics, such as morphine. Many anti-inflammatory medications (which we discuss later in this section) also relieve pain.

Among the most commonly prescribed analgesic medications that have no anti-inflammatory actions are codeine, drugs derived from codeine, narcotics, and synthetic narcotic compounds. These medicines include paracetamol with codeine, oxycodone, and dihydrocodeine.

 Always try regular over-the-counter paracetamol for your pain before using anti-inflammatories or prescription analgesics. Painkillers are strictly for pain relief. Use these medicines only for a short time unless your doctor has other reasons for suggesting long-term use.

In most cases, you can expect your doctor to prescribe analgesics only in the early phases of your acute back or neck pain. Doctors generally prescribe a time-limited course of pain medication along with other methods of pain relief such as limited bed rest, ice, and heat. You usually take analgesics on an as-needed basis. If you're experiencing short-term acute back or neck pain, analgesics may help – but don't wait until the pain is unbearable before taking the medicine. At that point, your pain may be so severe that the medication does little to help. And that means that you need more medication to get the pain under control. As this pattern repeats, you may find yourself experiencing higher levels of pain overall while actually taking more pain medicine.

If your doctor prescribes strong analgesics on a long-term basis, take them on a *time-contingent schedule* rather than as needed. In a time-contingent schedule, you take your medication on a fixed schedule – perhaps every four hours – regardless of your level of pain. This approach keeps the pain-relieving effects of the medicine constant and avoids the ups and downs of the as-needed approach. Time-contingent medication scheduling can help prevent severe pain episodes by 'catching' the pain early. In addition to using a time-contingent schedule, use the lowest level of pain medicine possible to stay comfortable. Doing so helps avoid tolerance and dependence and keeps side effects to a minimum.

Used correctly, pure narcotics are quite safe and have minimal side effects in *limited use*. You may experience dizziness, trouble focusing your thoughts, constipation, sedation, and lethargy, but these side effects tend to go away after a week or two.

Addiction

Research shows that when analgesics are taken for a legitimate pain problem, addiction to the drugs is rare. With appropriate use, narcotics are a safe and effective way to control your pain.

Opioid-based medications (narcotics) are one of your doctor's primary weapons against moderate to severe back and neck pain. The fear of addiction may cause you to avoid or even refuse these narcotics. Because of this fear, you may end up not taking adequate doses to provide relief or waiting to take the medicine until you can't bear the pain. To ease these fears, you need to understand the difference between tolerance, dependence, and addiction:

✔ **Tolerance** is a well-known property of all narcotics. Over time, your body gets used to the medication's effect, which sometimes means that you have to increase the dose to maintain effectiveness.

✔ **Dependence** is also a well-known physical process. If you suddenly stop taking the medicine, you may experience physical withdrawal symptoms, such as diarrhoea, agitation, and abdominal pain.

✔ **Addiction** is a *psychological craving* for the medication even when you don't need it for pain relief.

Your doctor can manage tolerance by adding other non-addictive medicines that help the narcotics work better and by using the other pain relief techniques that we discuss in this chapter. Your doctor can manage dependence by slowly tapering the pain medication (adding other medication to control withdrawal) when the time is appropriate.

Anti-inflammatory medications

Anti-inflammatory medications reduce inflammation. (How's that for a statement of the obvious?) Aspirin is probably the most common *non-steroidal anti-inflammatory* medication. In addition to reducing inflammation, aspirin and most other non-steroidal anti-inflammatories also help relieve pain. A number of different types of anti-inflammatory medication are currently on the market – common anti-inflammatories include ibuprofen and naproxen sodium.

These medications are standard treatments for back and neck pain, especially if your pain is possibly due to an inflammatory component such as muscle sprain–strain or injury to the soft tissues. Your doctor may also recommend anti-inflammatories for other spinal problems, including degenerative disc disease, arthritis, and disc herniations.

Your doctor may well prescribe anti-inflammatory medication on a regular dosing schedule, which allows the medicine to establish and maintain a therapeutic level. Plan to take the anti-inflammatory medication for approximately two weeks, unless your doctor instructs you otherwise. Resist the temptation to stop taking the anti-inflammatory medication when you start to feel better after a couple of days (unless your doctor tells you to stop) because you may actually start to feel worse. As with all the other medications, use anti-inflammatories in conjunction with other treatments for your back or neck pain.

Be aware that you may bruise more easily when taking anti-inflammatories because these medicines make your blood clot more slowly. Other side effects include ringing in your ears, light-headedness, and stomach upset. You can help avoid nausea and gastrointestinal upset by taking anti-inflammatories with meals. Contact your doctor if you have any of these side effects.

If you use anti-inflammatory medications for a long period of time (more than two months), you may be at risk of developing kidney and liver problems and peptic/gastric ulcers. When you've taken anti-inflammatories for an extended period of time, ask your doctor about other options. Avoid drinking alcohol when taking anti-inflammatory medications, because alcohol can increase the risk of bleeding ulcers.

Muscle relaxants

When your doctor believes that a muscle spasm or tightness is contributing to your pain, he or she may prescribe muscle relaxant medication. We believe that muscle relaxants are appropriate only when muscle spasm is clearly a prominent feature of your back or neck pain.

In addition to relaxing your muscles, muscle relaxants calm anxiety and agitation because of the way they affect your brain. Don't come to rely on these medications for their emotional calming effects.

No one knows exactly how muscle relaxants work. One theory is that the muscle relaxants operate on your brain and then secondarily on the muscles of your back. Alternatively, the medication may also act directly on the muscles themselves.

Among the more common muscle relaxants are methocarbamol and diazepam. Your doctor may prescribe the medications on an as-needed basis. Use these medications in conjunction with other techniques for reducing muscle tension and spasm, such as ice, heat, stretching, and biofeedback (Chapter 13 covers biofeedback).

Unless your doctor has a specific reason for prescribing muscle relaxants over a long period, take these drugs for a maximum of two weeks. In the initial stages of your pain, your doctor may prescribe these medications to help you sleep at night. This treatment needs to be short-term because these medications have a tendency to disturb healthy sleep patterns in the long run. In addition, long-term use of muscle relaxants can promote depression.

Common side effects of muscle relaxants include sleepiness during the day, difficulty with co-ordination, and depression, so avoid driving and operating machinery if you can. Avoid alcohol when you're taking muscle relaxant medications, as it can worsen these side effects.

Sedatives

When you're having trouble sleeping, your doctor may prescribe *sedatives* (also known as *hypnotics* – 'you're getting verrry sleeepy'). Before you use sedatives, discuss your sleep problem with your doctor.

- ✔ If your sleep problem relates to depression, a sedating antidepressant may be more appropriate than a sedative.

- ✔ If your sleep disruption is due to pain, an evening dose of a pain medication may be more appropriate.

Use sleeping medication only on an as-needed basis and for as short a time as possible. For long-term improved sleep, focus on other techniques such as relaxation training. Practise *good sleep hygiene*, which is not sleeping with a bar of soap but creating good sleep habits including:

- ✔ Go to bed and wake up based on a consistent schedule.

- ✔ Don't nap during the day.

- ✔ Do stressful things – such as paying bills – somewhere other than your bed or bedroom if possible.

- ✔ Get up if you don't fall asleep after 30 minutes. (You can try again when you feel more tired.)

When choosing a sedative, try the least addictive first. If your insomnia is due to pain, ask your doctor about trying paracetamol before taking prescription sleeping tablets. If paracetamol is ineffective, ask your doctor about trying a prescription medication such as a benzodiazepine (like diazepam or nitrazepam). Barbiturates have fallen into disfavour because of their potential for abuse and the availability of much safer medications.

Any sedative is to be used only when you need it and for as short a time as possible. Use the smallest dose that is effective in helping you to get to sleep. Although you can experiment with what works best for you, generally take the medication about 30 minutes before bedtime so that you're drowsy and ready to fall asleep when you hit the sack. The most common side effects are difficulty getting up the next morning (hangover) and sleepiness during the daytime. Do not drink alcohol when taking sedatives.

Anti-anxiety agents

When your back or neck pain is acute and associated with anxiety and trouble sleeping, your doctor may prescribe an anti-anxiety medication. Benzodiazepines such as diazepam and lorazepam are widely used anti-anxiety agents.

You may notice that we mention some of these medications in the preceding section. Medicines can fall into more than one category of use depending on their properties. Many of the anti-anxiety agents (and the antidepressants, which we discuss in the next section) are also good for sleep. Take these medications for a very short time when anxiety, specifically, is making your pain worse, and use these medications in conjunction with other treatment approaches. If, along with your back or neck pain, you're prone to anxiety or panic attacks, consider working with a psychiatrist or other doctor who has special expertise in prescribing anti-anxiety medications.

Common side effects of anti-anxiety medicines include drowsiness, sedation, and short-term memory loss. You can eliminate many of these side effects by working with your doctor to adjust the dose of the medications. Be aware that tolerance and dependence may develop when using these medications. (See the sidebar 'Addiction' in this chapter.) Avoid drinking alcohol with these medications. Never abruptly stop taking benzodiazepines or attempt to adjust the dosage yourself. Stopping these drugs abruptly can cause agitation, anxiety, sleep disruption, and, rarely, seizures: Instead, taper off these medications under your doctor's guidance.

Antidepressants

Antidepressants are becoming more and more common in the treatment of chronic pain problems. Extensive research now confirms that certain antidepressant medications can actually provide you with some pain relief, even when you're not depressed.

Even though your pain is felt in your back or neck, that pain is actually *experienced* in your brain. For this reason, researchers believe that the effect of antidepressants on certain chemicals in the brain provides not only an antidepressant benefit but also pain relief. Antidepressant medications appear to be particularly helpful in nerve pain problems and chronic pain.

Your doctor's choice of antidepressant medication for you depends upon your specific pain problem and associated symptoms. Some of the antidepressants have sedating properties, whereas others have more of an energising effect. In addition, different antidepressants affect different brain chemicals (such as serotonin and noradrenaline). Your doctor takes all these factors into account when choosing an antidepressant for you. You may need to try two or three different antidepressants before you find the one that works best for your situation.

The sedating properties of some of the antidepressants can be helpful in normalising sleep patterns, while at the same time helping to reduce your pain. Antidepressants seem to provide more restful sleep than do sedatives, along with other positive benefits such as pain relief. Antidepressants also help with the depression commonly associated with chronic back and neck pain.

As you can see in Table 8-1, the dosage ranges for pain relief and antidepressant effects are quite different. Even so, considering that depression is about four times more prevalent in people with chronic pain than in the general population, these medicines are certainly appropriate if you have significant depression with your ongoing pain.

Table 8-1	Dosage Ranges for Antidepressant Medications Used for Pain and Depression	
Antidepressant	*Dose for Pain*	*Dose for Depression*
Elavil	10–150mg	150–300mg
Molipaxin	25–75mg	150–400mg
Motival	25–100mg	75–150mg
Sinequan	10–100mg	150–300mg
Tofranil	25–75mg	150–300mg

Some other antidepressants, including fluoxetine, sertraline, and paroxetine, are also being studied for their effects on pain.

Antidepressants are usually effective only after they reach a certain level in your blood. If your doctor prescribes an antidepressant, you must take the medication every day (at bedtime or in the morning, depending on the drug) in order to reach and maintain that effective level.

Antidepressants vary in their side effects, but the most common include a dry mouth, blurred vision, constipation, difficulty urinating, sedation, and nausea. These side effects frequently occur in the first week or two that you take the antidepressant medication. If you can tolerate the side effects during this time period, they may then go away. When side effects are causing problems for you, talk to your doctor about other options. Antidepressants are not addictive, and you don't develop tolerance to them. You may need to take antidepressants for three to twelve months or longer. As with all medications, use other techniques at the same time for your back or neck pain, such as psychological pain management, counselling, relaxation procedures, meditation, biofeedback, and exercise – all may ultimately become substitutes for antidepressants.

Investigating Invasive Conservative Treatments

Invasive conservative treatments are treatments in which your practitioner pierces your skin. These treatments are still considered 'conservative' because they are reversible. Doctors usually reserve these treatments for patients whose back or neck pain doesn't respond to non-invasive conservative treatments. In this section, we first discuss the most common (and least invasive) invasive conservative treatments, before moving on to the less common (and more invasive).

Trigger point injections

A *trigger point injection* involves injecting a small amount of anaesthetic into certain muscle points, or *trigger points*. Your doctor may give you trigger point injections when you seem to have areas of muscle that 'trigger' pain throughout a region of your body such as your lower or mid-back. For instance, you may be able to point to certain specific areas in your back or neck that, when pushed with your finger, seem to cause pain not only in that local area but also throughout an entire region of your spine.

We recommend that you undergo trigger point injections on a time-limited basis, such as a few weeks or during flare ups of your back or neck pain, and only in conjunction with an overall active rehabilitation programme. Your doctor may recommend acupuncture instead.

Facet joint injections

If your doctor thinks that your pain is coming from your facet joints (see Chapter 3), he or she may recommend *facet injections*. These injections use steroid or anaesthetic to decrease the inflammation of the facet joint and provide pain relief. These injections are usually done on an outpatient basis in a centre with special radiology equipment called *fluoroscopy*. This equipment allows your doctor to see exactly where the injection is going into the facet joint. You may not notice the full benefit of a facet joint injection for at least one week after the injection, although you may get immediate relief from the anaesthetic (which then, unfortunately, wears off). Facet injections are given up to three times and at intervals at the discretion of the doctor giving them.

Spinal epidural steroid injections

In a *spinal epidural steroid injection*, your doctor – usually a rheumatologist or a pain clinic anaesthetist – injects steroid and sometimes an anaesthetic into an area (or *epidural space*) around the space in your spinal canal that contains the disc and spinal nerves. The steroid helps decrease inflammation and pain. Your doctor may recommend epidural injections if some type of disc or nerve root irritation problem is contributing to your pain.

Epidural injections are often done in a series of three. Most doctors don't give more than three epidural injections per six-month period because too much steroid in your spine isn't a good thing. Whether you have more than one epidural injection depends on your response to the first and the amount of steroid used. Research suggests that the full benefits of an epidural injection may not occur for up to ten days.

Agree to epidural injections when your doctor has a good medical reason and in conjunction with an overall exercise-oriented rehabilitation programme. We use epidural injections quite often on our patients with back and leg pain (sciatica) due to disc herniation. They can be extremely helpful in relieving pain and inflammation long enough to avoid surgery and allow natural healing to occur.

Selective nerve root blocks

Selective nerve root blocks are similar to spinal epidural steroid injections but are directed more specifically to the exact source of your pain. Selective nerve blocks shouldn't be performed without fluoroscopy (which we explain in the section 'Facet joint injections' earlier in this chapter) and are often diagnostic and therapeutic. They can be more effective than spinal epidural steroid injections in some cases.

The steroids used in selective nerve root blocks and spinal epidural steroid injections aren't going to make you look like Arnold Schwarzenegger. These steroids aren't anabolic (muscle-building) steroids; they reduce inflammation of the disc or nerve root.

Implantable pain therapies

Implantable pain therapies are the most invasive of the conservative treatments. Implantable pain therapies consist of two different types: spinal column stimulation and intraspinal drug infusion therapy. Both of these procedures involve minor surgery to place the devices in your body. Even though implantable therapies involve minor surgery, they're considered conservative because the treatment is reversible. These devices don't cure the problem but are designed to relieve your symptoms.

Consider these treatments only after you exhaust all other treatments for your pain without adequate benefit.

Implantable pain therapies aren't always a good idea. Therefore, your doctor needs to complete a screening evaluation (which we discuss next) that helps determine whether implantable pain therapy can work for you. Don't consider these treatments if any of the following items apply to you:

✔ Your symptoms don't match your physical findings, suggesting that the problem is not straightforward.

✔ You have depression and/or anxiety that clearly contribute to your back pain or leg pain.

✔ You show any signs of drug addiction or other problems, including a pattern of using pain medicines for purposes other than pain or not as prescribed by your doctor.

✔ You aren't motivated to combine implantable pain therapy with appropriate treatments to address other aspects of a chronic pain syndrome, such as exercise, psychological pain management techniques, and decreasing pain medication use.

✔ You have psychological or emotional factors (such as severe depression, anxiety, or other psychological problems) that may hinder a successful response to these types of treatments.

The preceding list includes some of the things that your doctor assesses as part of your screening evaluation. In addition, your screening includes a history to determine the reason why your other treatments didn't work, a physical examination to evaluate your pain, a psychological evaluation by a doctor familiar with pain problems, and a trial of any conservative therapy that hasn't been tried previously and your doctor thinks may be useful.

So few patients fit the criteria that few doctors ever use this treatment. That said, assuming you do have a condition that implantable therapy can help, and you pass the medical and psychological screening criteria, you may be a candidate for this type of treatment.

Spinal column stimulation

Spinal column stimulation was developed more than 30 years ago to manage chronic pain. In simple terms, *spinal column stimulation* involves surgically placing a set of electrodes along the nerve fibres of your spinal cord in your lower back, in order to block pain signals going through that area. The idea behind this treatment is similar to the rationale we discuss for TENS (see the section 'Transcutaneous electrical nerve stimulation (TENS)' earlier in this chapter). Your doctor may use spinal column stimulation as a last resort for failed back surgery syndrome, arachnoiditis (see Chapter 3), and nerve root injuries that haven't responded to other treatments.

Although first implemented more than three decades ago, spinal column stimulation didn't begin to gain popularity until recently due to technological advances. The increased success of this treatment is due to the use of new equipment making the surgery much less invasive, more durable parts of the implanted unit, computer technology that allows the power source to be tiny (similar to a pacemaker for your heart, the entire assembly is easily implanted, self-contained, and under the skin), and much better outcomes as a result of improving patient selection.

You may be an appropriate candidate for spinal column stimulation if you have the following characteristics:

- ✔ Your pain is primarily in one or both legs. Spinal column stimulators are generally not appropriate if lower back pain is your only complaint.

- ✔ Your symptoms and spine condition are stable and neither worsening nor improving.

- ✔ Your pain is due primarily to a nerve problem and radiates from your lower back to your legs.

- ✔ Your pain is primarily a burning, stinging, tingling, or radiating sensation.

- ✔ You have tried conservative treatments (such as physiotherapy, psychological interventions, nerve blocks, medication management, and multi-disciplinary rehabilitation), and they haven't helped.

If you're a possible candidate, your doctor places a temporary electrode to determine whether you can receive a permanent device. The test phase for the temporary electrode is approximately two to three days, although some surgeons require a test phase of up to two months. Your surgeon also requires anywhere from a 50–70 per cent reduction in pain with the temporary electrode in order to consider permanent placement.

You must be truthful with your physician as to the amount of pain relief you actually experience during the test phase. No matter how high your hopes, if the device doesn't work for you during the test phase, it isn't going to work after being permanently implanted, and you'll have undergone an unnecessary procedure and a treatment failure. The latest research indicates that about 50–60 per cent of qualified patients (those who meet the entry criteria) can expect greater than 50 per cent pain relief with permanent implantation of the spinal column stimulator. Complications of spinal column stimulation treatment are relatively infrequent and insignificant.

Intraspinal drug infusion therapy

If you have chronic pain due to failed back surgery syndrome or some other reason, and your pain has been unresponsive to any previous treatments, you may be a candidate for intraspinal drug infusion therapy. This treatment's primary use is for chronic, intractable, lower back pain.

Intraspinal drug infusion therapy involves surgically implanting a pump system in your body that delivers pain medicine by a small tube directly to a specific area of your spine. The rationale behind this approach is that you need much less pain medicine when the medicine is delivered in small quantities directly to your spine (actually about 1/300 of the same dose taken by mouth). When you take pain medicines orally, the results and effects occur throughout your entire body, and only a small portion of the medicine actually works where you need it. The intraspinal drug infusion method is designed to make the medicine more effective and have fewer side effects.

The screening criteria for an intraspinal drug infusion device are similar to those for spinal column stimulators, which we discuss in the preceding section. Other criteria that may lead your surgeon to choose this method over a stimulator include the following:

- ✔ Your pain is primarily in your lower back and buttocks with only minimal radiation down one or both legs.
- ✔ You have multiple pain sites in your lower back and buttocks.
- ✔ You don't describe your pain primarily as nerve root pain (refer to Chapter 2).
- ✔ You haven't responded to all other available conservative treatments such as medications, physiotherapy, nerve blocks, and psychological interventions.

After meeting all the preceding criteria, you undergo a test phase before your doctor considers a fully implantable pump system. In the test phase, you wear a pump outside your body that delivers pain medicine to your lower spinal area. The test phase lasts for one to three days, and you must notice at least a 50 per cent increase in pain relief. You must be truthful about the pain relief during this test phase because it accurately predicts the success of the permanently implanted device.

The permanently implanted system involves placing a small reservoir and pump under your skin. The pump has a tube that delivers the pain medicine to your lower spine. You need to refill the reservoir with pain medication at least every 90 days, although you may require more frequent refills. Refilling is a relatively painless procedure that is done at your doctor's surgery by placing a needle through your skin into the reservoir.

Complications related to intraspinal drug infusion devices include infection, contamination of the pump reservoir, cerebral spinal fluid leak, headache, mechanical pump failure, catheter failure, and side effects to the medication. Most of these complications are minor and reversible.

Chapter 9

Choosing to Have Surgery

- -

In This Chapter

▶ Recognising whether and when you need spinal surgery

▶ Getting the most out of your surgical consultation

▶ Understanding the different types of spinal surgery

▶ Preparing for back or neck surgery

- -

*W*e have some great news and some good news. The great news is that spine surgery is almost always your choice – yes, *your* choice. Only about 1 per cent of all spinal operations are truly medical emergencies, which means that approximately 99 per cent are elective.

Even if your doctor recommends surgery, most of the time you can safely opt to try a different treatment method first. Throughout this book, we offer you many alternatives for a more conservative, non-surgical approach to your back or neck pain. You may very well be able to manage your back or neck pain without surgical treatment.

Now the good news: In some instances, spinal surgery *is* your best bet to improve your pain. In fact, in our practice, we see a better than 90 per cent success rate with surgery due to our careful selective process and other techniques, which we review in this chapter. And because surgery is usually elective, you have time to prepare – something we also discuss in this chapter.

This chapter helps you decide whether to undergo surgery for your back or neck pain, shows you how to get information about your consultant surgeon, and gives you pointers for preparing for surgery. We also discuss some of the most common spinal operations.

We realise that some of the information in this chapter is frightening – surgery usually is. But we believe that the more you understand about the procedures and their inherent risks, the better equipped you are to decide whether to have spinal surgery. In our practice, we treat surgery as a last resort. In this chapter, we give you the tools to make the best choice for you and your back and neck.

Choosing to Have Surgery

Spinal surgery is almost always elective, unless you have an emergency condition such as the cauda equina syndrome, a spinal tumour, progressive neurological deficits, or a spinal infection (see Chapter 3 for more on all these conditions).

You may think that undergoing spinal surgery is a straightforward decision based on your medical needs: You may also think that spinal surgeons generally agree on what conditions are appropriate for surgery. However, the definitions of surgical and medical needs are as numerous as the surgeons who perform spinal operations. Whether or not your doctor recommends spinal surgery depends on two main factors:

- **Your symptoms and test findings:** As we discuss in Chapters 3 and 7, your findings from tests such as MRI scans must match your symptoms. That is, what the tests find and is therefore indisputable tallies with what you feel. Otherwise you have an increased risk of surgical failure. A doctor shouldn't consider surgery without being confident that he or she has identified the condition causing your pain.

- **The country you live in:** The rate of spinal surgery is much higher in the United States than in other industrialised countries, including the United Kingdom. Even different regions of countries have different rates of surgery.

Determining When Surgery Is Necessary

Occasionally spinal surgery is medically necessary, but usually surgery is *elective* – that is, you *choose* to have the operation. In this section we help explain the difference between conditions for which spinal surgery is your only option and conditions for which surgery is only one of several alternatives.

Medically necessary spinal surgery

Spinal surgery may be medically necessary if you have one of the following conditions:

- **Cauda equina syndrome:** In this extremely rare condition, important nerve roots in your lower spine, critical to the function of your bowels and bladder and responsible for sensation to your groin and anal areas, are compressed, usually due to a herniated disc.

Symptoms of the cauda equina syndrome include numbness in your genital and anal regions and in your feet, inability to urinate, and loss of sexual function. Without quick surgical treatment, you may lose permanently your bowel, bladder, and sexual function.

Having a disc herniation doesn't necessarily mean you have cauda equina syndrome. If your surgeon mentions the possibility of cauda equina syndrome, try asking the following questions:

- What is the likelihood that I have the cauda equina syndrome? (Remember that the condition is extremely rare.)

- What symptoms do I look for?

- What do I do if those symptoms occur?

✔ **Spinal tumour:** Even though spinal tumours may be non-cancerous and slow-growing, they may press on important parts of your spine, especially if you have a tumour in your neck or mid-back area. A spinal tumour may produce pain that wakes you up at night, and/or you may be more comfortable sleeping sitting up in an upright position on the bed.

If you have a slow-growing, non-cancerous spinal tumour that is not pressing on any important spinal areas, you may not need surgery.

Only a spinal surgeon can make a proper recommendation regarding the management of a spinal tumour.

✔ **Spinal infection:** Just as in any other part of your body, you can get an infection in your spine. You may be more vulnerable to spinal infection when your immune system is weakened (for example, if you're taking immunosuppressants) or you have diabetes.

Pain from a spinal infection is usually an intense, throbbing ache. The pain is often present when you are resting and may wake you up. Your doctor may diagnose a spinal infection on the basis of the results of your imaging tests, bone scans, and blood tests. Your doctor may be able to treat your spinal infection with intravenous antibiotics, but some patients need surgical treatment to clean out the infected area of the spine.

Elective spinal surgery

As we say elsewhere in this chapter, in most cases *you* choose whether to have spinal surgery. Your surgeon begins the process by suggesting that you're a candidate for surgery. You may be drawn to the quick-fix appeal of surgery, but we almost always tell our patients to avoid surgery if their back or neck pain is improving. You have no guarantee that surgery is going to improve your pain any better than a conservative approach and the natural course of healing (which we discuss in Chapters 6 and 8).

Because most spinal surgery is elective, you have time to make an informed decision. Consider the following issues in your surgical decision-making process:

- **You have leg pain rather than back pain.** Many doctors recommend spinal surgery to treat a disc herniation (see Chapter 3 for more on this condition) if your symptoms include pain in your buttocks, one or both legs, and/or your lower back. A herniated disc can take 12–16 weeks to heal, but 85–90 per cent of people are treated effectively without surgery. The herniated portion of a disc is mostly water, so the piece of disc causing the problem tends to shrink and be reabsorbed by your body over time. As the disc heals and shrinks, the irritation or pressure on the nerve is relieved and you feel better.

  If you have a lower-back problem that is appropriate for surgery, your symptoms are likely to include pain down one or both legs because the nerves that supply your legs pass through your lower back. You can have a lower-back problem, such as a disc herniation, without actually having any symptoms in your lower back.

- **You haven't responded to conservative treatments.** Conservative treatment (which we talk about in Chapter 8) is always an option. But if conservative treatment hasn't worked for you, a surgical approach may be appropriate. You may also consider surgery if conservative treatment has been only partially successful. Before you agree to surgery, give your conservative treatment enough time to work.

  Using only passive therapies such as hot packs and ultrasound (which we discuss in Chapter 8) is not an adequate course of conservative therapy. Active therapy is more appropriate.

  Even if your conservative therapy isn't entirely successful, surgery is still *your* choice. We have patients with residual symptoms, such as leg pain, numbness, and back or neck pain, who decide to live with these symptoms rather than resort to spinal surgery. These symptoms aren't dangerous, and as long as they don't worsen living with them over the long-term doesn't cause any problems.

- **Your symptoms match your test findings.** Spinal surgery can be highly successful if your doctor establishes clearly the reason for your pain through testing and your symptoms correspond to those results. For instance, if you have sciatica or leg pain due to a disc herniation, your pain is likely to be in a very specific area of your buttock and leg and matches your imaging studies and other diagnostic test results.

- **You refuse to accept the symptoms.** If your symptoms are worsening despite using appropriate conservative treatment, and you find the symptoms unacceptable, you may consider surgery.

Factoring risks

If you don't address emotional and psychological conditions before undergoing surgery, your operation may be a technical success but a clinical failure. An example is a patient who has surgery for a disc herniation: The post-operative MRI looks normal (*technical success*) but the patient continues to have debilitating pain (*clinical failure*).

The medical community is only now beginning to understand the power of emotional and psychological factors on surgical success. One study demonstrated how childhood psychological trauma influenced spinal surgery outcomes. The study looked at 86 patients who underwent spinal surgery as adults but experienced between zero and five psychological risk factors as children. Psychological risk factors included physical abuse, sexual abuse, abandonment, and emotional neglect or abuse. The study looked at the following points to assess the outcome of spinal surgery:

- Whether further surgery was necessary
- Results of an MRI of the spine six months after surgery
- Continued use of pain medication more than six months after surgery
- Inability or failure to return to work

As the number of risk factors increased, the probability of a successful outcome from surgery decreased. The probability of a successful outcome for a person with zero risk factors was 95 per cent. If a patient had four risk factors, the probability of a successful outcome was 7 per cent. A person with five risk factors had zero per cent probability of a successful outcome.

Addressing Psychological Issues and Surgery

Your surgeon may recommend surgery based solely on the physical aspects of your problem, including an MRI scan and other diagnostic test results (which we describe in Chapter 7), a physical examination, and your overall medical condition.

A good doctor also takes into account your psychological and emotional health. Some psychological and emotional issues may increase your risk of an unsuccessful outcome of surgery. As you prepare for surgery, make sure that you address any of the following issues that apply to you:

- **Depression, anxiety, or other emotional problems:** Address any depression or anxiety before considering spinal surgery.
- **Lack of support from family members or significant stress in family relationships:** Lack of emotional support can cause problems with the

entire surgical process. This kind of stress in your environment may also make your back or neck pain worse, which means that you may not make a well-informed decision about surgery.

✔ **Fear of pain or hospitals:** If thinking about post-operative pain or the hospital environment gives you the willies, talk to your doctor about ways to help you prepare for surgery (see also the section 'Preparing for Surgery' later in this chapter).

✔ **Negative surgical experiences:** A bad surgical experience can certainly make you nervous about going through another operation. Have a look at the section 'Preparing for Surgery' later in this chapter for help.

✔ **Unrealistic expectations:** Talk with your doctor about what you can reasonably expect from the operation. If you have unrealistic expectations, you may be dissatisfied with the results of your operation.

Ask your doctor or a mental health professional for help if any of the above points apply to you.

Some of our patients actually decide to forego surgery after dealing successfully with their emotional issues.

Some doctors believe that back or neck pain causes emotional issues and that surgery to fix your physical pain makes your emotional issues go away. Unfortunately, ongoing emotional and psychological issues affect your perception of pain and level of suffering. Surgery can repair a structural problem in your spine, but your psychological factors may continue and so may your pain.

Other factors can also influence the outcome of your spinal surgery. These factors include the following psychological and social issues (listed here in order of most common to least common):

✔ **Chronic pain syndrome:** The more symptoms of chronic pain syndrome you have (see Chapter 3 for a list of symptoms), the less likely you are to respond positively to spinal surgery. Treat all the elements of your chronic pain syndrome simultaneously. If you respond adequately and show improvement, you may not need surgery. Fixing a structural spinal problem with surgery but without addressing the other issues of chronic pain syndrome almost invariably causes a *failed back or neck surgery syndrome*. This is surgery that has not only failed but is itself the cause of additional pain.

✔ **Compensation and litigation issues:** Compensation and litigation issues, such as disability benefits and lawsuits relating to your back or neck pain, can cause psychological stress that affects your surgical outcome. If you're engaged in litigation related to your back or neck pain, or get compensation for it, you're at greater risk for a failed spinal surgery. This doesn't mean that you aren't a surgical candidate, but that you may have another risk factor requiring pre-surgical assessment.

✔ **Drug use:** If you take high levels of pain medication or other drugs, you risk having a poor surgical outcome, especially if you use your pain and disability as an excuse to abuse pain medication, other drugs, or alcohol. You also may have other non-physical risk factors such as depression or anxiety. Seek treatment for your drug abuse first, and then reassess the surgery option.

Getting a Consultation with a Spinal Surgeon

If you develop a medically critical condition requiring urgent surgical referral, your GP may refer you directly to a spinal surgeon. In the vast majority of cases, however, your GP or other doctor (see Chapter 4 for more on the professionals involved in your treatment) refers you to a consultant surgeon because your conservative methods of treatment have failed. To find out more about your spinal surgeon, follow some of the suggestions we make in Chapter 4.

A good surgeon shows compassion, explains your various treatment options, and discusses with you your reasons for choosing a particular kind of surgery. Your surgeon may not have time to answer pages and pages of questions, but you can expect your surgeon to allow you some time to ask questions. During your first one or two consultations with your spinal surgeon, try to get an idea of what your surgeon recommends and ask some general questions, such as the following:

✔ What is my diagnosis, and what does it mean for me?

✔ What is the natural pattern of my problem if we don't treat it?

✔ What are my treatment options?

✔ What are the risks and benefits of these options?

✔ Why do you recommend this specific course of treatment?

If you decide to have surgery, ask the following questions:

✔ What does the surgery entail?

✔ What are the possible complications, and how do you treat them?

✔ How am I going to feel after the surgery?

✔ How long am I going to be in hospital?

✔ What is my recovery and rehabilitation going to be like?

✔ What preparations can I make to ensure that the surgery is as successful as possible?

Understanding the Different Types of Spinal Surgery

In this section, we discuss some of the most common types of spinal surgery. We start with the least invasive surgery and move on to more invasive operations.

Chymopapain injection or chemonucleosis

If you have disc herniation and related sciatica (leg pain), your surgeon may suggest *chemonucleosis*. In this outpatient procedure, done under local anaesthetic, your surgeon injects an enzyme called chymopapain into your affected disc to dissolve some of the disc. You have only a local anaesthetic during this surgery because both you and your surgeon need to be aware if the needle touches a nerve so that the needle can be redirected. Before chemonucleosis, your surgeon makes sure that you're not allergic to chymopapain by testing a small amount on you.

The risks of chymopapain injection are:

✔ Infection

✔ Allergic reaction to chymopapain, which vary from a local reaction to a general reaction

✔ Paralysis due to a reaction to the enzyme, which can lead to weakness of one or both legs

Doctors can't predict with certainty the risk of paralysis following chymopapain injection, and chemonucleosis is therefore rarely used in the UK.

The success rate for relief of sciatica following chymopapain injection is 65–80 per cent in patients who meet the stringent inclusion criteria.

Percutaneous discectomy

In *percutaneous discectomy*, your surgeon removes a portion of your disc using a laser or suction device. During this outpatient procedure, you are awake under general anaesthetic in order to avoid nerve injury during placement of the probe into your disc (because you'll feel the probe touch a nerve – ouch!). The surgeon uses *fluoroscopy*, a special type of X-ray, as a guide to place the probe properly. Some surgeons also monitor the probe *arthroscopically* (using an endoscope). After percutaneous discectomy, you can usually return to sedentary types of work and limited activities after 48–72 hours.

Percutaneous discectomy may be appropriate if you have sciatica (leg pain) due to disc herniation or you have intermittent severe attacks of lower-back pain associated with *scoliosis*, a condition in which a disc herniation causes a severe spasm in the muscles on one side of your spine resulting in curvature of your spine.

 Percutaneous discectomy is a low risk procedure, but it can cause disc space infection or injury to a blood vessel or nerve. Some patients' symptoms recur three to six months after the procedure, permanently at times. We feel the usefulness of this procedure for treating sciatica is limited and conservative treatment is often a better choice.

Microsurgical discectomy

In *microsurgical discectomy*, your surgeon partially removes some of the disc causing the symptoms and a small amount of the bone covering the spinal canal through an incision less than 2.5 centimetres (one inch) long and using a microscope (see Chapter 2 for more information on spinal anatomy). You're likely to be in hospital for one day. The procedure is done under general anaesthesia and takes from 45 minutes to several hours, depending on how much work needs to be done.

As with any spinal surgery, we suggest you try conservative treatment before agreeing to microsurgical discectomy. You may consider microsurgical discectomy in the following situations:

✔ You have a herniated disc with sciatic (leg) pain.

✔ You have progressive neurological loss, such as weakness, causing you significant problems in daily functioning.

✔ You are elderly and have *spinal stenosis* (a narrowing of the spinal canal) associated with a disc herniation, which is causing sciatic pain.

✔ You have a recurrent disc herniation.

You're likely to be walking around the morning after surgery. You shouldn't experience a great deal of pain after this operation and any pain you do have can usually be controlled with appropriate pain medication. The local discomfort from the surgery usually goes away within several days. However, the sciatica can take some time to disappear, depending on how long the nerve was irritated before surgery and how long the nerve takes to recover, a process that can take up to two to three months or longer.

The risks of microsurgical discectomy include infection, injury to the nerve root, a bad reaction to anaesthetic, blood clots, and recurrent disc herniation. In order to prevent infection, your surgeon gives you intravenous antibiotics during the operation. Infrequently, the nerve root is manipulated during surgery, which can cause numbness and/or weakness in the nerve distribution – this side effect sounds frightening, but usually goes away after a week or so.

Your surgeon removes only the portion of your disc that is irritating or compressing the nerve root. As some of the disc remains, you have a small chance of recurrent herniation. If re-herniation occurs, you may experience a sudden recurrence of your sciatic pain after being free of pain. Unfortunately, this pain may be much more intense than your original sciatica. If conservative treatment fails, repeat surgery is almost always successful.

Laminectomy

During a *laminectomy*, your surgeon first removes the *lamina* (the back part of the vertebra) and then the associated ligament to remove your herniated disc. Removing the herniated disc alleviates the pressure and/or irritation of the affected nerve roots.

Your surgeon may use laminectomy to take pressure off the spinal canal when you have *spinal stenosis*, a narrow spinal canal. If you have recurrent, residual problems from a previous operation (such as local scarring or deformity), your surgeon may recommend laminectomy to remove some additional bone, which makes more room for the nerves.

You're likely to be in hospital for two to five days. If you're elderly, you may need extra time for rehabilitation and recovery and may need to stay in an extended-care facility for several weeks. Complete recovery takes four to six months – sometimes even longer – but you can start physiotherapy approximately two to three weeks after the operation.

The risks associated with laminectomy are similar to those for microsurgical discectomy (which we discuss earlier in this section). However, the risks are greater with laminectomy due to the longer operating time and because it is quite a major procedure.

Spinal fusion

A *fusion* is an operation in which your surgeon attempts to stop the movements that normally take place between two adjacent vertebrae. Sometimes, a spinal fusion involves the use of *instrumentation* or *fixation devices* such as metal rods, screws, or *cages* (small cylinders placed between the vertebrae). Spinal fusion technology changes rapidly, so we give only an overview here. Three main types of spinal fusion are used:

✔ **Posterior fusion:** Most fusions use the *posterior approach* (that is, from the back). In this procedure, the surgeon removes part of the bone of the two vertebrae, and then places fresh bone, taken from your *iliac crest* (pelvic bone) or hip, in your back with the aim that these elements eventually grow together. As the vertebrae grow together, they form one solid unit with almost no movement between them. Screws and rods can enhance fusion rates and allow you to be more active, sooner.

✔ **Anterior fusion:** The surgeon makes an incision near your belly button to access the front of your spine. Anterior fusion may make use of fixation devices called cages. If you undergo this very complex procedure, we believe that a spinal surgeon and a general or vascular surgeon need to do the surgery together whenever possible. A team of different surgical specialists increases the operation's safety.

✔ **Combination fusion:** Rarely, surgeons do both a posterior and an anterior fusion. You may require both types of fusion when previous operations have failed, you smoke (see the sidebar 'Smoking and spinal fusion'), or you have had complications such as infection. In these cases, you have two separate surgical procedures, under a single anaesthetic or several days apart.

Spinal fusions are much less common than disc excisions. Surgeons primarily recommend fusion to alleviate *mechanical* lower-back pain (pain made worse by activities such as bending, twisting, and lifting is usually alleviated by rest) when X-rays show some kind of instability between two vertebrae.

Even though spinal fusion involves significantly greater risks than the other operations we discuss in this chapter, the risks are still quite low. The risks of spinal fusion include the following:

✔ The fixation device may fail or break.

✔ The hip area, from where the bone graft is obtained, may cause pain.

✔ The vertebrae may fail to grow together.

Weigh the risks and benefits when you consider spinal fusion surgery. This major surgery is associated with considerable time off work and rehabilitation. We believe that you should rarely have fusion for sciatica due simply to a disc herniation.

Smoking and spinal fusion

When you smoke, you face a serious risk with fusion. Smokers have significantly less chance of a successful fusion (as low as 60 per cent compared with 85 per cent of non-smoking patients). If spinal fusion fails, the bones of your back don't grow together as they should.

We recommend you stop smoking for a minimum of four to six weeks before surgery and then make every effort to not smoke until your fusion is firmly united as well. And if you stop for that long, you may as well not start smoking again!

Preparing for Surgery

We divide preparing for spinal surgery into medical, psychological, and psychosocial aspects. Most surgeons focus on the medical aspects of the surgery and exclude the other two areas. However, considering all three areas increases your probability of a successful outcome.

Medical preparations for surgery mean reviewing the medication you're taking. Based on your doctor's advice, stop taking aspirin, drugs that contain aspirin, non-steroidal anti-inflammatories, and blood-thinning medications for at least three to ten days (depending on the medicine) before your surgery. These medicines may increase bleeding, leading to complications during or following the surgical procedure. Your doctor should direct and monitor this process.

Psychological screening and preparation for surgery can be important, especially when you've had an unsuccessful operation before or are having an extensive operation. In these cases, we recommend that you have a pre-operative psychological evaluation from a psychologist skilled in the evaluation and management of chronic pain problems. Your surgeon may recommend you undergo a brief psychological preparation programme with a clinical psychologist (your surgeon refers you). Such a programme gives you the opportunity to discuss your anxieties and fears, your expectations of the surgery, and the predicted course of your treatment. Make sure that your surgeon gives you plenty of information about what to expect before and after your hospital stay. You may consider trying relaxation training (which we describe in Chapter 13) or pain and anxiety control.

Psychosocial preparation for surgery may include the following:

✔ Planning for your absence from, and return to, work.

✔ Resolving insurance and financial issues.

> ✔ Anticipating your return to a more active lifestyle, including exercise.
>
> ✔ Preparing your family for your post-operative rehabilitation.

If you're elderly, you may need to arrange to stay in an extended-care facility after surgery before you return to your own home.

Try to engage in normal activities until the time of your surgery, and use this period to address any predictable problems (listed above) before your surgery.

Looking at the Future of Spinal Surgery

Spinal surgery has changed dramatically over recent years and changes are likely to continue. If you had lower-back surgery for a disc herniation several years ago, your surgery involved an incision several centimetres long, a hospital stay of between four days and a week, and two to three months before you returned to your normal activity.

With the advent of keyhole surgical techniques, surgeons can now do this operation through a 2.5–4 centimetre (1 to 1½-inch) incision. You stay in hospital for only one night and then return to normal light activities within two to three weeks.

The developments for lower-back surgery have a bright future. Researchers believe that spinal surgical incisions are going to get even smaller. In addition, more advanced instruments are going to help spinal surgeons to work even more accurately within the small confined space of your spine.

Another exciting development may be performing spinal surgery within an MRI scanner. This technique gives your spinal surgeon a continuous update on how the surgery is going. MRI technology may also allow your surgeon to revise the procedure during the operation as necessary.

Part III

Complementary Approaches: Are They for You?

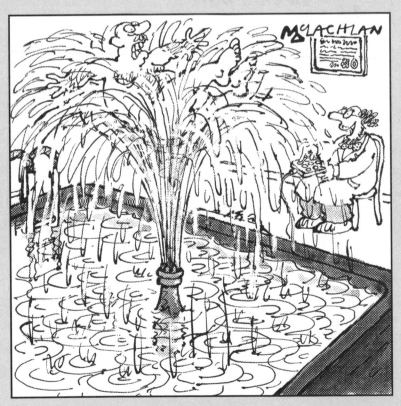

"It's a new type of hydrotherapy
– Let me know when you've had
enough, Mr Maybrick."

In this part . . .

You may find yourself drawn to non-traditional back pain treatments. We believe that these complementary approaches can work very well under the right circumstances – especially when you combine them with the traditional options that we discuss in Part II of this book.

Complementary approaches sometimes get a bad name. Although they're not a panacea, they may help you, and you are the important one here. This part takes a look at some of the common complementary methods, including chiropractics and yoga, among others.

Chapter 10

Ancient Eastern Wisdom and Contemporary Ideas

· ·

In This Chapter

▶ Finding a complementary medicine practitioner

▶ Picking the right complementary approach

▶ Discovering different complementary treatment approaches

· ·

*P*eople are looking increasingly towards complementary medicine approaches for relief from a variety of health problems, including back and neck pain. Some people abandon conventional treatment altogether, but others supplement conventional medical treatment with alternative measures.

When working with back and neck pain, we prefer the term *complementary medicine* rather than holistic or alternative medicine, because this term promotes the idea of conventional medical approaches to back and neck pain working in concert with complementary medical interventions. We don't like to think of complementary medicine approaches as being alternative to standard medical treatment. In our opinion and in the way we practise, the most powerful approach is to combine the two orientations in an appropriate manner.

In this chapter, we help you pursue complementary medicine treatments in a safe manner and avoid treatments that may harm you. We discuss the general issue of selecting a complementary medicine practitioner. Then we focus on some of the complementary medicine approaches commonly used to treat back and neck pain.

Appendix B can guide you to finding a suitable complementary medicine practitioner.

Selecting a Complementary Medicine Practitioner

When you're seeking an expert in complementary medicine, try using many of the same criteria you use to select a conventional doctor. The following list offers some basic guidelines for choosing a complementary practitioner:

- **Choose a generalist with a diverse background.** Find a practitioner with a diverse background and expertise in a wide variety of areas. We often recommend finding someone who can use both complementary and conventional medicine treatments. This practitioner is more likely to be able to balance his or her approach in a rational manner.

  When seeking treatment with a complementary medicine practitioner who specialises in one approach, make sure that the treatment is co-ordinated with your conventional physician.

- **Find a practitioner with whom you can establish a good rapport.** As with any practitioner, you want to feel comfortable with your complementary medicine practitioner. A good relationship with your practitioner includes open communication and an overall sense of trust in the person's abilities.

- **Rely on a referral source that you trust.** One of the best ways to find a good practitioner is through a referral, from your doctor or from someone the practitioner has treated. Talking to someone you trust who's had experience of the practitioner can give you a good idea about the practitioner's bedside manner and conduct.

- **Select a practitioner sensitive to your needs.** Find a practitioner who has experience of treating back and neck pain and attending to any requirements specific to your case, such as associated symptoms.

- **Beware of practitioners who aren't willing to work with your doctor.** Successful treatment of conditions such as chronic back and neck pain often involves a collaborative effort by a variety of different professionals. If any practitioner is unwilling to work with other disciplines you've found helpful, take this refusal as a warning sign.

This advice includes not only complementary medicine practitioners but also your GP. Your doctor needs to be willing to discuss complementary medicine approaches with you in a non-judgemental and open fashion. Your GP may not agree with certain complementary medicine approaches, but he or she can still help you make an informed decision about pursuing this type of treatment. For example, if you're interested in osteopathy, your doctor may advise that you consult a registered osteopath.

> ✔ **Don't rely on credentials alone.** A degree, medical or otherwise, isn't an automatic guarantee that a complementary medicine practitioner's recommendations are safe. Develop a trusting relationship with the practitioner, but also investigate any recommended treatments yourself.

Choosing the Best Complementary Medicine Approach for You

In complementary medicine, the mental and emotional aspects of healing must be dealt with in conjunction with the physical. Even if the complementary medicine approach you choose seems to focus primarily on the physical, you still need to be mentally and emotionally comfortable and confident in the treatment. This section helps you evaluate complementary treatment methods before taking the plunge.

Asking the right questions

After you decide to try a type of complementary treatment approach, try to identify a practitioner or two with whom you may be interested in working (based on the guidelines we describe in 'Selecting a Complementary Medicine Practitioner' earlier in this chapter). Ask the practitioners the following questions to help you choose wisely among the complementary treatments available for your back or neck pain:

✔ How long has this treatment been available?

✔ How commonly is this treatment used for back or neck pain, and in what percentage of back or neck pain cases has this treatment been documented to be successful?

✔ What risks and potential side effects are associated with this treatment?

✔ Are any other treatments better or more effective, and would they achieve the same result?

✔ At what point in the treatment do I know if the treatment is working?

✔ What is a reasonable treatment trial, for example how many sessions may I need?

Avoiding quackery

To have a positive experience with complementary medicine, you need to avoid being treated by a *quack* (a practitioner who performs a treatment or service without having the necessary knowledge, skills, or qualifications).

The following guidelines can help you identify quackery:

- ✔ **Beware of quick fixes:** Quacks often claim that their treatments can produce immediate cures. When you have chronic back or neck pain, you may be more susceptible to claims for a quick fix due to your frustration over the ongoing pain and your longing for relief.

- ✔ **Beware of anecdotal evidence:** Testimonials and case histories are often used to support claims for a particular treatment that allegedly cures a condition such as back or neck pain. These testimonials often target conditions that conventional medicine has found difficult to treat. Chronic back and neck pain fall into this category. Even when patients have given the testimonials sincerely, any number of factors other than the complementary medicine approach may explain dramatic improvements. These factors include the natural improvement or fluctuation of the pain over time and the *placebo effect* (getting better because you expect to improve).

- ✔ **Beware of secret formulas:** The active ingredients of any medicine must be disclosed on the label. Pharmaceutical companies must publish reports listing the ingredients of their drugs and explaining how they work. You should expect the same approach to labelling for any product that claims to have a medicinal benefit. Avoid any products that don't list their contents.

Considering Specific Complementary Treatment Methods

Complementary medicine offers many treatment options for back and neck pain. The following sections describe some of the treatments commonly used to treat back and neck pain.

Acupuncture: Needling your way to a better back and neck

Acupuncture is one of the most common complementary medicine approaches used to treat back and neck pain. Acupuncture – which has been practised in China for more than 5,000 years – is a complete system of healing based on the ancient Chinese theory of *qi* (also referred to as *chi* and pronounced 'chee').

Traditional Chinese theory on acupuncture

According to traditional Chinese acupuncture theory, *qi* is the vital life energy present in all living organisms. Qi circulates in the body along 12–14 major energy pathways called *meridia*. These meridia are on each side of the body and criss-cross along the arms, legs, torso, and head, and deep within the tissues. Each meridian is believed to link to a specific internal organ and organ system.

The meridia surface at different locations on the body called *acupuncture points* or *acupoints*. Traditional acupuncture theorists and researchers believe that hundreds to thousands of these acupoints exist within the meridian system and can be stimulated to enhance the flow of qi. This stimulation causes healing. Special needles placed just under the skin at specific acupoints provide the necessary stimulation to correct and rebalance the flow of energy. Opposing forces within the body, called *yin* and *yang*, must be in balance before the qi can get your vital functions (spiritual, mental, physical, and emotional) to work normally. This stimulation of the acupuncture points provides pain relief and healing properties.

A contemporary Western take on acupuncture

Not surprisingly, the ancient Chinese explanation of acupuncture differs markedly from the theory that Western medical researchers propose. Western researchers typically dispute the existence of qi and provide different explanations for the effects of acupuncture. They believe that stimulating an acupuncture point causes the release of endorphins in the brain and other helpful natural chemicals in the body. *Endorphins* are naturally occurring substances in the brain that cause a decreased perception of pain. Research supports this theory, showing that when animals or humans are given naloxone, a chemical that blocks the action of endorphins, the effects of acupuncture are stopped.

In addition to rejecting the concept of qi, many Western scientists don't accept the existence of a separate independent system of meridia. Instead, they point to studies demonstrating that acupuncture points, when viewed under a microscope, show a greater concentration of nerve endings than other skin locations. According to this view, acupoints are part of the nervous system rather than an independent system.

Many Western physicians are critical of acupuncture and believe that its effects are simply a *placebo response* – responses attributed simply to the patient's *belief* that the treatment is going to work. No matter what the explanation, the release of endorphins has been proven in humans after acupuncture.

A typical acupuncture treatment programme

At your initial consultation, the acupuncturist is likely to ask you to complete a questionnaire regarding your medical history and your back or neck pain.

The acupuncturist then investigates symptoms not typically addressed by Western medicine. For example, the practitioner may take a very close look at your tongue, which is considered in acupuncture to be a primary source of diagnostic information. Other areas that the practitioner may assess include the tone of your voice, your body language, the colour of your urine, your menstrual cycle, your sensitivity to temperatures and seasons, any digestive problems, your pulse, your eating and sleeping habits, and your emotional status.

After the initial evaluation, with your agreement the acupuncturist places special acupuncture needles in the appropriate acupoints. Acupuncture needles are extremely thin and vary in length from a fraction of a centimetre to several centimetres. These needles are usually made from surgical stainless steel, but sometimes they are made from gold, silver, bamboo, or wood.

Although most acupuncturists use disposable needles, always check to make sure that your acupuncturist uses only sterile disposable needles.

Depending on your condition, an acupuncture treatment involves using up to 10 or 12 needles placed at specific locations. As the needles are placed in the acupoints, the practitioner may gently twist them by hand for 15–20 minutes. The twisting is thought to alter the chi and help the treatment. You may feel a dull heavy sensation when the chi (or the nerve) is stimulated. This is normal.

The placement of the needles is generally painless. Patients tell us that they experience a slight pricking sensation when the needles are inserted. The competence and experience of the acupuncturist relates to the amount of physical sensation that you may notice.

Tell the acupuncturist if you feel any discomfort as a result of needle placement. Sometimes, the acupuncturist needs to change the needle position or pressure slightly, which can eliminate the discomfort you're experiencing.

You may notice that the needle placement doesn't necessarily correlate with the location of your pain or symptoms. This discrepancy is based on the theory of meridia, which we explain in the section 'Traditional Chinese theory on acupuncture' earlier in this chapter. The practitioner may place needles in your ears, head, face, legs, arms, or torso, and all may be nowhere near the place where you're experiencing symptoms.

The needles are generally left in for 15–30 minutes, but in certain instances, depending on the individual practitioner, this period can be longer. Many, but not all, our patients report a temporary feeling of heaviness or a slight ache at the location of needle treatment.

Other approaches to stimulation of acupoints

Acupuncturists also use other means of stimulating acupoints. A common technique is to apply heat by burning a herb called *moxa* (mugwort) above the acupoint to be treated. Chinese studies suggest that this herb is unique in its ability to stimulate the acupoints and facilitate the body's self-healing abilities. The acupuncturist burns a very small amount of moxa on a slice of ginger placed on top of an acupoint. In some cases, the moxa is placed and burned directly on the acupoint and then removed when the patient reports the temperature is too warm to tolerate further.

Another traditional treatment for areas of large muscle pain is *cupping* with a glass or bamboo cup. The acupuncturist puts the inverted cup over the painful area. The cup creates a suction area on the skin over the painful area.

The number and frequency of sessions depends on your problem and on the competence and beliefs of the practitioner. In our experience, some patients respond in a few sessions with long-lasting benefits, some have a good initial response but require periodic maintenance treatments, and some experience no benefit at all. If you notice no benefit after the first 6–12 sessions, you're unlikely to benefit from further treatment.

Effectiveness of acupuncture for back and neck pain

We believe that acupuncture is most effective when included as part of a comprehensive treatment approach. Your acupuncture plan may be complementary to a conventional medical intervention and/or in conjunction with other complementary medicine approaches, such as taking appropriate exercise and making healthy lifestyle changes.

The effectiveness of acupuncture and its mechanism of action are controversial in scientific communities. Scientists have difficulty separating the mechanical effectiveness of acupuncture from the patient's belief that the treatment is going to work. However, this problem exists with many other medical approaches as well, and in our clinical practice, we don't see this issue as particularly important: When you have a positive response to the treatment, and little risk is involved, the reason for your response doesn't really matter.

For more information about acupuncture, check out the resources listed in Appendix B.

Appreciating aromatherapy

Aromatherapists believe that *essential oils* (the fragrant essence of plants) contain the life-force of the plants from which they are extracted. In aromatherapy, this life-force is absorbed through the skin or inhaled to stimulate the body's tissues, promote healing, and restore the balance between mind, body, and spirit.

Essential oils are highly concentrated substances, so they are used in tiny amounts, diluted with a much larger amount of *base* or *carrier oil* (other plant or fat oils such as almond oil). Essential oils are believed to have painkilling, antiseptic, and anti-inflammatory properties and to be able to improve the function of the immune system by making it more effective. Many oils have more specific healing qualities: Some are particularly recommended for people with back or neck pain, such as bay laurel, eucalyptus, ginger, and marjoram.

A typical aromatherapy treatment programme

You can apply the oils on a compress, in a bath, or inhale them. However, having a massage is believed to be the most effective form of aromatherapy for back and neck pain.

At your initial consultation, you're given an initial assessment, and then the therapist applies the oils to the painful area. Each consultation usually lasts an hour.

Effectiveness of aromatherapy for back and neck pain

No reliable scientific evidence exists to support the effectiveness of aromatherapy in back and neck pain, but many people find it extremely helpful, in relieving or reducing back or neck pain.

If you are pregnant, take great care with aromatherapy: Always seek treatment from a qualified therapist, don't use aromatherapy in the first three months of pregnancy, and avoid aromatherapy altogether when your pregnancy has complications.

If you have a history of allergic skin reactions, discuss aromatherapy with your GP before you seek aromatherapy treatment, as you may be sensitive to essential oils. Other than these warnings, aromatherapy is harmless and has no side effects.

Taking up t'ai chi

T'ai chi is an ancient Chinese system of physical movement designed to harmonise the individual with the forces of nature. The graceful, slow, flowing movements of t'ai chi are thought to integrate the forces of yin and yang within the body, creating the balance essential for health and wellbeing, both physically and spiritually. As this balance is achieved, the *qi*, or life-force (which we describe in 'Acupuncture: Needling your way to a better back and neck' earlier in this chapter) is able to flow correctly through the body and the individual becomes harmonised with the universe and everything in it.

Practising t'ai chi regularly is believed to improve flexibility and fitness, speed up recovery from injury and illness, help prevent further illness, and relieve depression and other psychological symptoms.

A typical t'ai chi session

In t'ai chi the back is kept straight and the head is held high in all the movements, actively ensuring good posture. You learn a series of separate movements that you then run together into a continuous sequence or form. You always carry out the movements in the same order, one movement naturally flowing from the previous one. The short form consists of about forty movements and takes about eight minutes to complete. The long form has over a hundred movements and can take more than half an hour. Learning the form takes a variable number of sessions, usually lasting up to an hour, either in a one-to-one session or as a class.

Effectiveness of t'ai chi for back and neck pain

People with back and neck pain often find that t'ai chi is an excellent therapy. The slow, flowing movements provide the benefits of Western aerobic exercise but without the stresses and strains that frequently cause injury. Little scientific evidence exists in favour of t'ai chi, but practising t'ai chi regularly seems to help weight loss, improve flexibility, and tone the muscles and ligaments supporting the spine and the rest of the skeletal system, which helps to protect against the recurrence of back and neck pain.

T'ai chi is unlikely to be harmful because it is so gentle.

Rebalancing with reflexology

Reflexology, or *reflex zone therapy*, is a special foot massage based on a system of energy pathways that run through the body. Reflexologists view the underside of the foot as a chart of the human body. They believe that the foot is divided up into different areas, or *reflex zones*, connected to specific organs and structures, such as the spine, shoulders, and head. Reflexologists maintain that illness is the result of energy imbalances in certain organs and body structures and that these imbalances are reflected in the corresponding area on the soles of the feet. By massaging these areas, a reflexologist can detect and then correct the problem, clearing the way for the body to heal itself.

A typical reflexology treatment programme

At your first consultation, your reflexologist makes an initial evaluation.

Reflexology sessions typically last up to an hour. The practitioner asks about your symptoms and then spends some time examining your feet. The reflexologist may identify problems at this stage if certain areas of your feet feel tender or sore.

The practitioner uses his or her thumbs to massage the tender areas of your feet. When you have neck pain, the reflexologist may press on the base of your big toes, as this zone corresponds to the neck. When you have back pain, the reflexologist may apply pressure to the inside edges of your big toes and along the inside of your feet, as this area corresponds to your spine.

The treatment may be slightly painful at first, but this sensation soon disappears as treatment progresses through the session and is often replaced by a feeling of relaxation and wellbeing. Reflexology has no known side effects.

Effectiveness of reflexology for back and neck pain

No agreed scientific theory exists as to how reflexology works, but many people report that the treatment eases back and neck pain and sciatica. Reflexology is not harmful.

Bodywork

The therapeutic use of touch has been used for centuries to heal the body and reduce tension. *Bodywork* refers to therapies such as massage, deep-tissue manipulation, movement awareness, and energy balancing. Bodywork is used to reduce pain, soothe injured muscles, stimulate blood and lymphatic circulation, and promote deep relaxation. Patients often seek some type of bodywork for help with their back or neck pain problems.

Hundreds of types of bodywork treatments are available. In this section, we review several well-established bodywork systems, with the aim of helping you find a style of bodywork that may be effective for your back or neck pain. Note, however, that we're dealing with professional bodywork and massage techniques, and not how to give a massage.

Some common elements of bodywork treatments include:

- ✔ **Pressure or deep friction** to move muscles, connective tissues, and other body structures.

- ✔ **Patient education and awareness** of posture and movement to improve physical functioning and pain.

- ✔ **Stretching, muscle balance, and relaxation** to improve physical functioning and reduce pain.

- ✔ **Breathing and emotional expression** to eliminate tension and enhance physical abilities.

Bodywork treatment for back and neck pain is highly variable in terms of the actual approach to treatment, the length and frequency of treatment the practitioner recommends, and the cost per session. As you investigate body-work treatment, use the list in 'Asking the right questions' earlier in this chapter to help you select a practitioner. As with all complementary treatment approaches, we recommend that you seek your GPs advice before working with a bodywork practitioner.

Many forms of bodywork include an approach developed originally by Dr Wilhelm Reich, a psychoanalyst and student of Sigmund Freud. Reich was one of the first people to state that your body's posture and behaviour reflect your feelings and emotions. He developed a system of bodywork and breathing techniques that he believed may bring buried emotions to the surface. Reich felt that bodywork decreased chronic physical tensions and released unconscious feelings and memories. Many practitioners of bodywork have incorporated Reich's techniques in order to address physical and emotional issues simultaneously.

For more information about bodywork, check out the resources listed in Appendix B.

Pilates

The *Pilates method* (often shortened simply to *Pilates*) is a system of physical conditioning developed by Joseph Pilates almost a century ago. Determined to overcome his childhood illnesses, Joseph Pilates studied Eastern and Western forms of exercise and developed special machines to help with his rehabilitation.

Pilates has a strong emphasis on proper body alignment, injury prevention, correct breathing, and muscle stretching and strengthening. Although professional dancers originally popularised the method, Pilates is appropriate for people of all ages, abilities, and lifestyles, including people with back or neck pain.

The goal of Pilates is to promote muscle elongation rather than build bulk – so you don't have to worry about turning into the Hulk. Pilates attempts to develop your abdomen and lower back into a firm *core* of support for your whole body. The programme promotes alignment, balance, and stabilisation of your spine, which, in turn, makes safely working other parts of your body easier.

Along with specific exercises on the floor, Pilates training may involve a *universal reformer*, which sounds like a device from Star Trek but is actually a low bench-like piece of exercise equipment that uses springs and ropes for resistance. You lie, sit, stand, or kneel on the movable platform and control a sliding carriage by pushing or pulling with your feet or hands on straps, bars, or pulleys. Your trunk muscles are the main focal point for each movement, and each movement is performed with breath, ease of motion, and relaxation.

Pilates is very different from other exercise approaches. Therefore, make sure that a professional Pilates instructor treats you.

Therapeutic massage

Massage is one of the most frequently used therapies for back and neck pain. Research indicates that therapeutic massage can have several beneficial effects on back and neck pain, including:

- ✔ Relaxing the nervous system and muscles
- ✔ Lessening scar tissue and lessening fibrosis and adhesions that develop as a result of injury
- ✔ Reducing swelling
- ✔ Improving blood flow through the muscles

Muscle tension from activity, injury, or stress may contribute to muscle fatigue and pain by pushing on nerve fibres in the muscle. Therapeutic massage releases muscle tension and promotes relaxation. Muscle *contraction* (tightening) for an extended period of time interferes with the elimination of chemical waste products in the muscles and surrounding tissues. The longer a muscle is tense, the more these chemical waste products build up and irritate the nerves and muscles in the area, causing more pain. Therapeutic massage can help break down these muscular waste deposits and stimulate more blood flow to the painful areas.

Alexander technique

Around the turn of the twentieth century, Frederick Matthias Alexander noticed that faulty posture – sitting, standing, and moving – during daily activities relates to physical and emotional problems. The *Alexander technique* uses awareness, movement, and touch to try to rebalance the body. The technique focuses on developing the correct relationship between the patient's head, neck, and back while engaging in proper (or natural) movements.

Classes in the Alexander technique usually last an hour at a time. The basics are usually taught over a series of about ten classes, and lessons are offered on a one-to-one basis. It is not painful and there are no contraindications or side effects.

Feldenkrais method

Moshe Feldenkrais was a physicist who suffered a sports-related injury. Instead of submitting to surgery to treat his injury, he studied the nervous system and human behaviour to find another solution. He applied his experience with martial arts, physiology, anatomy, psychology, and neurology to develop his own treatment programme. Feldenkrais was able to reverse his impairment and walk without pain.

The *Feldenkrais method* focuses on improving your self-image, changing negative habitual patterns of movement, healthy breathing, and functioning with greater ease, fluidity, and motion. The approach encourages you to explore and experiment with movement in order to find your own optimal style of movement. In addition, the practitioner may actively direct your movements by using touch.

Rolfing

Ida Rolf was a biochemist, first exposed to therapeutic manipulation when an osteopath successfully treated her for a respiratory condition. As a result of her treatment, Rolf began to develop the primary tenet of her treatment approach: The structure of the body affects all physical and psychological processes. Rolf was also influenced by her exposure to yoga. She established the Rolf Institute in 1970.

Rolfing is based on the idea that human function improves when the body is aligned properly. Rolf believed that if your body is out of alignment, your muscles are over contracted and stressed. After maintaining this unhealthy posture for months or years, other tissues in your body have to compensate to hold everything in this out-of-balance position. Movement becomes impaired, which in turn reduces your mental clarity and increases emotional stress.

During Rolfing, the practitioner manually manipulates and stretches the body's fascial tissues to re-establish the patient's balance. The *fascia* is a thin elastic membrane that surrounds every muscle, bone, blood vessel, nerve, and organ. The practitioner applies pressure to the fascia using his or her fingers, knuckles, and elbows. This treatment can cause mild to significant pain depending on the amount of pressure applied. In addition to the physical manipulations, Rolfing includes education about movement.

Chapter 11

Chiropractic and Osteopathic Solutions for Your Back and Neck Pain

· ·

In This Chapter

▶ Understanding chiropractic and osteopathic approaches

▶ Deciding when to use chiropractic or osteopathy

▶ Getting a grip on diagnosis and treatment methods

▶ Knowing when to end treatment

· ·

*C*hiropractic and osteopathy have long been popular complementary therapies for back and neck pain. We cover the two therapies in one chapter because they have a good deal in common.

Both chiropractic and osteopathy have statutory regulations, meaning that all chiropractors and all osteopaths have undergone similar standards of training, are covered by professional indemnity insurance, and adhere to professional codes of practice. The approaches and methods of diagnosis of chiropractic and osteopathy are quite similar – both disciplines have spinal manipulation as the keystone of their therapeutic activity.

Chiropractic and osteopathy now have more scientific respectability than they were once shown. In view of this growing acceptance, medical guidelines for the management of back pain state that when the pain lasts for more than a few days chiropractors, osteopaths, physiotherapists, and doctors who have been trained to manipulate the spine can really help by being involved in the person's treatment. Sadly, treatment is rarely available on the National Health Service.

Understanding the Chiropractic and Osteopathic Ways of Thinking

The core philosophy of the chiropractic approach is that your body has the inherent capacity to heal itself. In this approach, the chiropractor helps you achieve health naturally. Chiropractors use a mechanical treatment known as *manipulation* or *adjustment* to correct the original mechanical injury, in an attempt to allow your body to resolve problems and heal itself.

Sometimes, however, the damage done by trauma or degenerative disease may be too severe for chiropractic alone. If that situation applies to you, seek additional help from a conventional medical doctor or surgeon.

Chiropractors agree that most back and neck problems begin with some type of injury to your spine or surrounding muscles. Injury can occur from a single event such as a car accident or from repeatedly using bad posture. The injury leads to a series of events that determine how you experience your back or neck symptoms. For instance, you may have symptoms that are close to the injury site, such as local back pain and spasm. Alternatively, you may have symptoms that are remote from the injury site, such as radiating pain to your arm or leg.

Chiropractors vary in the attention they pay to possible emotional and psychological contributions to back and neck pain. Some chiropractors focus only on structural explanations for your back or neck symptoms and plan their treatment accordingly. Others focus on both mind and body influences on your symptoms.

Osteopaths regard the body as an integrated unit and believe that a problem in any area can have a knock-on effect, causing dysfunction and pain elsewhere. For example, osteopaths believe that when a misaligned vertebra puts pressure on nearby nerves, the result is dysfunction of various internal organs and the glands that produce the body's hormones. According to this view of the human body, once the misalignment in the spine is corrected, the body can heal itself.

Choosing Chiropractic or Osteopathy

Manipulation is a safe and effective method for dealing with various types of pain, although some types of pain respond better than others. For example:

✔ **Acute back pain** is most likely to benefit from manipulation.

✔ **Radiating pain** travelling down your legs may be more difficult to treat, but manipulation is still worth a try.

✔ **Chronic pain** may benefit from manipulation. Manipulation may not make your pain go away totally, but it will certainly help to keep it in check and reduce the number of recurrences you have.

Sometimes, the tissue injury from trauma or degenerative disease may be too severe for manipulation to help. If your pain isn't relieved in a reasonable amount of time (a week to 10 days), your chiropractor or osteopath may suggest you consult your conventional medical doctor.

Before you choose a chiropractor or osteopath, ask a few questions:

✔ **What problem are you treating me for?**

Your chiropractor or osteopath should tell you what he or she thinks is causing your pain. Your practitioner should also explain the activities of daily living that you need to avoid and those activities that may be helpful for your condition.

✔ **How long before I feel an improvement?**

Most patients feel some temporary improvement immediately. A few people have local soreness after the first treatment for a day or less (try using ice to relieve the soreness). Most people feel a lasting improvement within two to four weeks.

✔ **What other treatments are available to me?**

Your treatment options depend on what's causing the pain and whether your pain is a recent or long-standing problem. Other treatment options may include drugs, massage therapy (which we talk about in Chapter 8), physiotherapy, and rehabilitation exercises.

✔ **What is the next step, if the treatment doesn't work as expected?**

During the first four weeks of treatment (if your pain lasts that long), your chiropractor or osteopath modifies your treatment specifically for you. If you feel no improvement in that time, your chiropractor or osteopath may suggest you see a conventional medical doctor for diagnostic tests. Your pain may respond best to treatment that includes both conventional medicine and chiropractic or osteopathy.

✔ **What can I do myself to improve my recovery?**

You can help yourself by recognising that although back and neck problems are an inconvenience – sometimes major – they usually don't seriously alter your enjoyment of life. Try to follow your chiropractor or osteopath's recommendations on restrictions and exercises. In general, walking, swimming, and bicycling may be helpful for your pain.

✔ **Are you going to speak to my GP or specialist about your findings and recommendations?**

Open communication and co-operation between your practitioners is the best way for you to get the treatment you need.

Knowing What to Expect

On your first visit, your chiropractor or osteopath is likely to ask about your health and medical history, how your back or neck pain began, and how the pain affects you now. Your chiropractor or osteopath may ask you to remove some of your clothing, down to your underwear, so he or she can examine you properly.

After making a diagnosis, your chiropractor or osteopath explains what he or she believes is wrong and then recommends a treatment plan. If you agree with the plan, treatment begins.

In addition to manipulation, your chiropractor or osteopath may suggest other things to speed up your pain relief, such as wearing a brace or corset, taking nutritional supplements, and exercises for you to do at home.

Making a diagnosis

First, your chiropractor or osteopath probably asks you how, when, and where your pain or symptoms occur. They rely heavily on examining you to determine the site of your problem and the best method of treatment, so he or she may then perform a physical examination. He or she may test your reflexes and ask you to perform some simple tasks, such as bending your back and limbs, contracting your muscles against resistance, and assessing skin sensation.

Chiropractors and osteopaths use their highly trained sense of touch (known as palpation) to assess the muscles and bones of your back, neck, or extremities to determine any tight muscles and tender areas. He or she may put the painful area through specific motions to test the integrity of your joint ligaments and other tissues, and apply light pressure to detect whether pressure makes your symptoms worse.

Some chiropractors recommend all their patients to have X-rays as a precaution. However, many patients with back or neck pain don't need X-rays or other extensive testing. We believe that X-rays are necessary only if your pain was brought on by injury, your examination suggests the possibility of a serious illness (such as a tumour or an infection), or you haven't healed as expected. Spinal X-rays aren't risk-free, so make sure that a good reason exists for having an X-ray. Chapter 7 talks about X-rays and other diagnostic tests.

Most back and neck pain don't require special tests. Always ask how the results of a special test may possibly change your treatment, because if it doesn't change your treatment, there's no point in having it done.

Your osteopath or chiropractor needs to build up as complete a picture as possible of you and your symptoms. He or she is likely to ask where in your body the problem started, where exactly you feel pain, whether the pain is permanent or intermittent, and what the pain feels like. In general, they take into consideration all aspects of the person's health and lifestyle (such as diet, occupation, and exercise) before making a diagnosis.

Your osteopath or chiropractor is likely to examine not only the painful areas of your back or neck but also the rest of your body. This approach is to determine whether problems elsewhere are causing or contributing to your back or neck pain. You may have problems in areas that you don't associate with your back or neck. They may check the movements of your joints and observe how your body responds to the normal demands of everyday life, such as sitting down, standing up, and walking.

Starting treatment

All chiropractors and osteopaths undergo manipulative treatment procedures as part of their training. Most chiropractors focus on joint manipulation of the spine and *extremities* (arms and legs).

After making a diagnosis, your osteopath is likely to use various manipulative techniques to try to correct your problem. These techniques include flexing, stretching, and massaging the spine, arms, and legs.

Your chiropractor or osteopath may also recommend exercises to do at home (work your way to Chapter 15 for more on exercising), ergonomic modifications for your home and office (which we explain in Chapter 16), supervised exercise therapy to rehabilitate your spine, and *nutrition counselling* (recommending that you eat or avoid certain foods or supplements) to promote healing.

If chiropractic or osteopathic treatment is appropriate for your pain, you experience improvement fairly quickly. When you've had your pain for more than three months or so, your improvement may begin slowly and gradually. In addition, you may not feel an improvement in all your symptoms at the same time.

Keep in mind the 'three steps forwards, one step back' rule: When treating people with back and neck pain, we often see patients move forwards – they feel better and become more active – before moving back a little. But if you move forward three steps and back one step, you're still two steps better than you were. Keep this concept in mind so you don't get discouraged when you have a setback or flare up of your pain.

Looking at the Side Effects of Manipulation

All effective treatments have possible side effects. Fortunately, manipulation is generally very safe, and the potential complications are minor. The most common side effect is soreness in the manipulated parts of your body after your first treatment. Other temporary symptoms include feelings of fatigue or warmth in your arms and legs. These complications are short-lived and leave no permanent effects.

Nerve damage and stroke are extremely rare complications of manipulations. These complications occur so infrequently that most chiropractors and osteopaths never see a single case in their entire career. To put things into perspective, the risk of having nerve damage or a stroke as a complication of manipulation is much smaller than the risk of developing an ulcer after using over-the-counter painkillers.

If you sometimes feel dizzy when you stand up or turn around, manipulation is not for you (see Chapter 2 for information about the vertebral arteries, that can make you feel dizzy when they block). Also avoid chiropractic and osteopathy when you have a condition that directly affects or weakens the bones or joints, such as rheumatoid arthritis, osteoporosis, or bone cancer. If in doubt, always consult your GP before seeking chiropractic or osteopathic treatment.

Stopping Manipulative Treatment

Your chiropractor or osteopath looks for a measurable improvement in your pain and function. Stop treatment when your symptoms are no longer improving or they're getting worse.

No one can predict how long effective treatment is going to take. Many people take less than eight weeks to heal with chiropractic or osteopathic treatment. We recommend trying between 6 and 12 sessions and then stopping treatment if you have no lasting improvement. If you do see continuing improvement, press on.

The following factors may mean your recovery takes longer:

- ✔ You've had your symptoms for more than eight days.
- ✔ You've had more than three prior episodes of the same problem.
- ✔ You have another problem in your bones or joints, such as arthritis, disc degeneration, or herniation.

We don't recommend spinal manipulation for a disk herniation with nerve compression, as the treatment may worsen the condition.

Chapter 12

All in Knots: Trying Yoga

*Y*oga is one of the oldest known systems of health. The breathing exercises, physical postures, and meditation practices of yoga can reduce your stress, regulate your heart rate, lower your blood pressure, and relieve your back or neck pain.

The word yoga means *union*. Yoga is the integration of physical, mental, and spiritual energies that come together to enhance your overall health and wellbeing. Patanjali was the first person to describe yoga systematically in *The Yoga Sutras* in the second century BC. Yoga says that if your mind is chronically agitated and restless, this anxiety negatively affects the health of your body. Alternatively, if your body is in poor health, your mental strength is drained.

Yoga is more than a few exercises – instead, it includes a complete system of lifestyle changes, hygiene, and detoxification methods. Yoga comprises both physical and psychological practices. You can find whole volumes written about yoga, and we can't present an entire yoga approach in just one short chapter. But you may want to check out *Yoga For Dummies* by Georg Feuerstein and Larry Payne , (Wiley).

This chapter offers advice on using yoga to relieve your back or neck pain. Appendix B suggests some places to head for more information about yoga.

Beginning Hatha Yoga

One of the most widely used yoga practices is *hatha yoga*. In hatha yoga, you complete a series of body positions and movements (*asanas*), which involve stretching and holding the postures, and breathing exercises (*pranayama*). These exercises can create almost immediate positive changes in your body that can help with your back or neck pain. The asanas and pranayama prepare you for meditation (which is called *samadhi* at its most advanced state), yet another aspect of yoga.

- ✔ Asanas bring your spine and head into alignment to promote proper blood flow throughout your body, and then bring your mind into a state of relaxation. Also, asanas help energise your lungs and heart. Many health care practitioners suggest yoga as part of the treatment for back, neck, and joint pain.

- ✔ Pranayama focuses on regulating your breath to promote physical relaxation, calm your mind, create mental focus, and increase your energy.

- ✔ Samadhi is an advanced level of meditation that comes from practising the asanas and pranayama. We discuss the nature of samadhi later in this chapter.

Practising yoga postures

Asana means 'ease' in Sanskrit. Even though many of the yoga postures, or asanas, involve little movement, the mind is actively involved in the performance of every asana. By practising yoga postures, you discover how to regulate automatic nervous system functions such as your heartbeat and breath and allow your physical tensions to relax. This process in turn can help relieve or even prevent back and neck pain.

The asanas are designed to balance opposites, such as forwards with backwards, stillness with movement, and inhaling with exhaling. One of the best known asanas is the *lotus position*. In the lotus position, your left ankle is on top of your right thigh and your right ankle on top of your left thigh, and the backs of your hands rest on your knees. But don't try this on your own: You need to work up to this level of flexibility under the guidance of a qualified yoga instructor.

Controlling your breath

Breath control, or *pranayama*, focuses on the way you regulate your breath. Pranayama literally means the regulation or control of *prana*, which is your life-force. An interruption in the flow of prana due to factors such as stress, improper diet, or toxins in your body, damages your physical, emotional, and mental health.

The alternate nostril breathing exercise

Alternate nostril breathing is a simple pranayama exercise that can help promote the flow of *prana* (the life-force) and promote relaxation.

Begin by sitting upright on a cushion or firm chair with your head, neck, and body aligned. Take three complete breaths focusing on breathing from your diaphragm. (We cover this breathing technique in Chapter 13, but basically this way of breathing involves filling your lungs from the bottom up rather than breathing only through your chest.) Make your inhalations and exhalations of equal length, slow, controlled, and smooth.

After taking three complete breaths, begin the alternate nostril breathing technique. First, close your right nostril with the thumb of your right hand and exhale completely through your left nostril. After you have exhaled completely, close your left nostril with your right index finger and inhale completely through your right nostril.

Repeat this cycle of exhaling through your left nostril and inhaling through your right nostril two more times. Make sure that you maintain an equal length of time for inhaling and exhaling. At the end of inhaling the third time through the right nostril, exhale completely through the same nostril while keeping the left nostril closed. At the end of this exhalation, close your right nostril and inhale through your left nostril.

Repeat this cycle of exhaling through your right nostril and inhaling through your left nostril two more times. Then place your hands on your knees while exhaling and inhaling through both nostrils evenly for three complete breaths. At this point, you have completed one cycle of the alternate nostril breathing exercise. The following is a summary of the entire exercise:

Complete breaths, both nostrils	Three times
Exhale left and inhale right	Three times
Exhale right and inhale left	Three times
Complete breaths, both nostrils	Three times

As you practise this technique, gradually lengthen the duration of your inhales and exhales. We recommend that you practise the alternate nostril breathing exercise at least twice a day, once in the morning and once in the evening.

Pranayama exercises promote the proper flow of prana throughout your body. The exercises help you focus your mind while bringing your breathing into a steady and rhythmic state. For a simple pranayama exercise, see the sidebar 'The alternate nostril breathing exercise'. As we discuss in Chapter 13, breathing exercises induce the *relaxation response*, which leads to benefits such as decreased heart rate, lowered blood pressure, reduced muscle tension, and lowered levels of pain. Breath exercises are often performed as a preparation for meditation.

Meditating towards samadhi

The asanas and pranayama can lead to a state of meditation in which your physical body is extremely relaxed and your mind is highly focused. The most advanced practice of meditation leads to spiritual realisation, or *samadhi*, which is the culmination of lengthy, dedicated, and disciplined practice. Those in the know describe samadhi as a different state of consciousness beyond the states of waking, sleeping, and dreaming.

The meditative state can be very beneficial, even if you never get to samadhi. When you're in a meditative state, you may notice a heightened sense of awareness and overall wellbeing. Meditation can reduce muscle tension, slow your heart rate, lower your blood pressure, improve oxygen consumption in your body, improve your immune function, and reduce pain.

Using Yoga to Treat Back and Neck Pain

Yoga can be very effective for your back or neck pain because it addresses several factors that may be making your condition worse. Yoga can help with your posture, strength, flexibility, weight and diet, and overall mind and body relaxation. One survey of patients with back or neck pain showed that 98 per cent of the people surveyed found yoga to be beneficial for their back or neck pain.

One of the common causes of back and neck pain is prolonged overstretching of the back and neck ligaments and muscles due to poor posture during sitting and standing. (For more about posture, check out Chapter 14.)

Most people bend forwards too much throughout their day. Improving your everyday posture when sitting, standing, walking, lifting, and sleeping can help with your pain – and even prevent pain from occurring in the first place. Poor posture takes its toll on your body – especially your back and neck – after days, weeks, and years of repetition. Poor posture causes chronic physical problems even in young people in their 30s and 40s.

Think about your average day: You wake up in the morning, sit on the edge of the bed, and bend forwards. You walk into the bathroom, use the toilet, and bend forwards. As you prepare for the day, you stand in front of the mirror and bend forwards, perhaps shaving or putting on make-up. You get into your car and bend forwards while driving to work. After arriving at work, you sit in a chair and bend forwards at your desk. Back at home, you may sit in your home office and bend forwards in front of your computer. All that bending forwards may be too much for your body.

A simple way to experience the effects of a prolonged stretch is to turn both palms up with your fingers extended. Push the tip of your left index finger down with the tip of your right index finger (right palm above left palm) while keeping the left palm and forearm parallel to the floor. At first you notice pressure at the end of your left finger; after a short while, however, you feel radiating pressure going down the entire finger, your hand, and eventually your entire arm. This process is exactly what happens to your back and neck ligaments and muscles during prolonged periods of slouched sitting or standing. Tension in one part of your body (for example, your back or neck) causes pain and tension in other areas as well.

At first, maintaining a healthy back and neck may sound like a full-time job. But with practice, the exercises we discuss in this book and techniques such as good posture, become second nature. When that happens, promoting a healthy back and neck becomes a lifestyle rather than an ordeal you have to think about all the time.

A weekly session or two of yoga or exercise therapy is not going to help much if you misuse and abuse your spine the rest of the time.

Yoga therapy can be an excellent approach for your spinal problem, by itself or as part of an overall treatment plan. Yoga not only helps to improve your posture and back or neck pain, but also enhances your entire life.

As with any complementary medicine treatment, we suggest you check with your doctor before starting yoga practice.

Using yoga exercises for your back and neck pain

If you have a serious back or neck problem that significantly interferes with your activities or limits your ability to exercise, consider initially working one-to-one with a yoga therapist. Choose a yoga therapist with experience of working with people who have back and neck pain, to alter some of the yoga movements to accommodate your back or neck pain. In addition, the yoga therapist may have you move through the exercises at a slower pace than usual in order to keep your pain under control as you discover the techniques.

Many classes exist that show you the general techniques of yoga. Although you may progress towards group classes, starting out with an individual yoga therapist may be the wisest choice. A group yoga class can be risky if you have a back or neck problem, especially when the class is large. To find a yoga instructor, start with the resources in Appendix B. Other good places to look are local community centres and health clubs. You may also find a dedicated yoga centre in your area – some even specialise in back and neck pain.

Although some nationally recognised yoga organisations exist (see Appendix B), getting a recommendation for an instructor from family, friends, or your health care professional can be more helpful. As you check out an instructor, consider asking to talk to some other satisfied clients.

One main goal of any good yoga or exercise programme for the back or neck is to restore the normal range of movement to your spine, including flexion (bending forwards), extension (bending backwards), and rotation (twisting). The challenge is to determine which type of programme you need and to inspire you to complete a daily exercise routine that fits your lifestyle and allows you to progress at a safe speed. Your yoga therapist and doctor can work together (or at least communicate periodically) to accomplish this goal and design a safe, maximally effective yoga programme for you.

The key to yoga exercises for your spinal problem is knowing what, when, and how much to do. Prescribing a particular yoga posture or programme for your unique problem is beyond the scope of this chapter.

In general, however, if you're like many people, you may suffer from weak abdominal muscles, tight hamstrings, and strained or sprained ligaments and muscles that support the curves in your spine. Additionally, if you have injured or had surgery on your spine, you may have scar tissue that needs to be stretched out in order for your spine to become functional again. A specific yoga exercise programme can help achieve these goals for your problem and bring your body into balance.

Keeping a daily journal

As we discuss in Chapter 15, getting an exercise buddy can keep you up to scratch by checking that you're keeping up with your exercises. Another idea is to keep a daily back or neck journal. Your journal can be long and complicated or very simple. Usually a simple journal is best, because you may shy away from anything that takes too much time. On a piece of paper or in a diary, keep track of the following information on a daily basis:

- Did you do your yoga or back or neck exercises today?
- Did you feel pain? If so, at what time of the day? Give the degree of pain a rating from 0 to 10, with 0 being no pain and 10 being the worst pain possible.

On another piece of paper, take a few minutes to record the activities during your normal day that cause pain in your back or neck. For example, 'My lower back hurts on the right side when I take out the rubbish' or 'My back hurts when I sit too long.' After a week or two of writing in the journal, review your entries and look for patterns. With this information you can better tailor your activities and yoga exercise programme to keep your pain under control.

You may find that taking short breaks throughout the day helps prevent a build-up of back or neck pain. You may also discover that doing a few yoga movements and breathing/meditation exercises throughout the day helps you break up the pain cycle. In addition, if you're having a particularly bad day, you may feel a lot better when you look back on your calendar and notice how many good days you've had. An occasional bad day is part of the normal healing curve – we always tell our patients to expect three steps forwards, one step back – so try not to get down.

Resting and Relaxing

When you don't get a good night's sleep, you invite more back and neck problems, as well as other poor health conditions. Many people don't understand that both the mind and the body need a rest. In our fast-moving society, getting your thoughts off work and other stressful matters is difficult. Just because you physically lie down in a bed for eight hours doesn't mean you're getting the rest you need.

Reducing your back or neck pain requires good sleep hygiene. Yoga breathing and meditation exercises can be an integral part of this programme. *Sleep hygiene* means that you take steps to ensure that you obtain a restful night's sleep. Examples include avoiding stressful activities in bed (such as working on your bank statements and watching the news), getting up after a half hour when you can't fall asleep, and avoiding coffee and energising activities such as exercise just before you go to bed.

What goes into your mind just before going to bed and while you're trying to fall asleep can affect your entire night's sleep pattern. Even though you may be physically asleep, your mind can be quite stressed. This anxiety results in a restless night's sleep that doesn't restore your energy for the following day. Symptoms of a stressful night's sleep can include clenching your teeth, waking during the night and not being able to fall readily back to sleep, and feeling tired the following day. Yoga breathing and meditative exercises can help you get a good night's sleep, which in turn helps your body and mind effectively fight off your back or neck pain during the day.

Chapter 13

Using the Power of the Mind–Body Connection

. . . .

In This Chapter

▶ Changing your thoughts to decrease your pain

▶ Practising relaxation and imagery

▶ Beginning biofeedback training

▶ Trying self-hypnosis

. . . .

Many factors – physical, mental, and emotional – influence your back or neck pain. As we mention throughout this book, you can have severe pain with minimal physical findings or minimal pain with severe physical findings. Your mind can influence your body in significant ways, including:

✔ Whether you experience certain types of back or neck pain, such as stress-related pain.

✔ Whether you heal from your back or neck injury or pain quickly.

✔ Whether you experience depression and anxiety as part of your back or neck pain.

Thoughts and emotions have a significant influence over your pain and you can use your thoughts and emotions to help make the pain better.

The term *mind–body connection* refers to how your mental and emotional states ('mind') affect your physical being ('body'), and vice versa. The connection works both ways (mind affecting body, and body affecting mind), but the focus is generally on your mind's influence over your body. The mind–body connection can work *against* you, making your pain worse, or work *for* you, helping you overcome your pain.

Mind–body techniques are becoming more popular. The techniques are useful for the management of many medical conditions, including back and neck pain. In this chapter we discuss the mind–body techniques of changing your thoughts and emotions, using relaxation and imagery exercises, biofeedback, and hypnosis. Mind–body techniques are often not labelled directly by the medical profession, but are utilised.

You need to practise mind–body techniques on a regular basis in order for them to be effective. Keeping yourself motivated is the most important component of successfully using mind–body approaches to improve your back or neck health. Motivation and practise can reward you with positive results such as improved health and less pain. You can help yourself stay motivated by rewarding yourself along the way, perhaps with that special something you've been after for ages.

Taking Control of Your Thoughts and Emotions

You constantly evaluate the world around you and the sensations going on inside your body. These thoughts are *automatic*: They tend to be very fast, *unconscious* (out of your awareness), and highly credible. But how can a thought be both unconscious and credible? Actually, you have unconscious, credible thoughts all the time. For instance, if you play golf and face a challenging shot, you may have the unconscious thought that you can't make the shot because you've missed it a few times before, even though consciously you tell yourself that you *can* make it. The unconscious thought can be highly credible, even though it remains unconscious, and causes you to foul up the shot. The evidence that you believe the unconscious thought is your emotional and physical sensations, such as self-doubt, anxiety, and trembling.

Automatic thoughts have a great influence over your emotions, behaviours, and pain. The good news is that you can recognise these negative automatic thoughts and change them into positive automatic thoughts.

Recognising automatic thoughts

Research shows that human beings under stress have a tendency to engage in irrational *negative* automatic thoughts. Negative automatic thoughts, as the term implies, tend to produce negative states and emotions such as depression, anxiety, and fear, and they can create increased pain sensations. Identifying when you're experiencing negative automatic thoughts and understanding how negative automatic thoughts work can put you on the road to changing those thoughts.

Having back or neck pain may be a stressful situation that can result in a variety of negative automatic thoughts, perhaps including some of the following:

- ✔ 'I'll never get better!'
- ✔ 'My back or neck is getting worse and worse!'
- ✔ 'I'm going to end up in a wheelchair!'
- ✔ 'Why is this happening to me?'

Not only is this type of thinking negative, but also – and more importantly – often these statements are inaccurate if you consider them carefully.

Almost all our patients with back or neck pain acknowledge having these types of thought at some time. Our patients also admit that these thoughts are highly credible when they occur.

You can probably guess the consequences of having and believing negative thoughts. Try reading out loud the thoughts in the preceding list. Simply by reviewing a list of negative statements, most people begin to feel sad and nervous. In fact, if you have back or neck pain, you may notice your pain worsening as you review and think about these statements. However, by challenging these thoughts and turning them around, you can feel better again, as we show in the next section.

Using automatic thoughts to your advantage

Coping, or rational, thoughts are directly opposed to negative automatic thoughts. *Coping thoughts* reflect the true reality of the situation and help you focus on the range of options available to help you solve a problem such as back or neck pain. Coping thoughts may be similar to the following:

- ✔ 'No one can predict the future, and I benefit more by being optimistic rather than pessimistic.'
- ✔ 'This pain doesn't mean that I'm getting worse. I'm showing improvement in the following ways . . .'
- ✔ 'I have no evidence that this back or neck pain is going to make me end up in a wheelchair.'
- ✔ 'I'm going to think about what I can do to improve my situation instead of spending my time asking why this happened to me.'

Each of these coping thoughts directly disputes an associated negative automatic thought from the list in the previous section. Try reading out loud the coping thoughts. Simply by reviewing these coping statements, you may begin to feel a little more hopeful and optimistic. We sometimes ask our patients to carry around a list of coping thoughts to review throughout the day.

You don't have to be a victim of negative automatic thoughts. Instead, begin to identify negative automatic thoughts as they occur and replace them with coping or nurturing thoughts. Be aware these negative thoughts can occur very quickly and you need to look at your train of thought to reveal the statements you've been telling yourself.

Changing your thoughts

Negative automatic thoughts can cause negative emotions such as anxiety, fear, and anger, which in turn can worsen your back or neck pain. In a vicious circle, your pain causes you more stress, resulting in an increasing cascade of negative automatic thoughts.

We recommend a useful model for understanding how your thoughts, emotions, and behaviours interact. You may find the *ABCDE model* a good tool for changing your thoughts and dealing with your back or neck pain. In the ABCDE model:

A is the *activating event* or *antecedent event*, which is the event to which you're responding. This event can come from outside, such as sitting in a traffic jam, or from inside, such as severe pain.

B is your *belief* or automatic thought about the activating event. For instance, your belief about your pain may be 'I'll never get better! My back or neck is getting worse and worse. I'll end up in a wheelchair!' On the other hand, your conscious thoughts about your pain may be 'This pain doesn't mean I'm getting worse. This is usually a temporary thing. I'm getting better overall. This pain is nothing to be frightened of.'

C is the *consequent emotion* resulting from your automatic thoughts. Most people think that the activating event causes this consequent emotion, but in reality your belief causes your emotion. Your emotional response to a situation is caused by your beliefs about the situation, not by the situation itself.

D is the *disputing thought* that you can use to change negative automatic thoughts. Disputing thoughts can help you change the way you think about a stressful situation, such as your back or neck pain, from a negative standpoint to a coping standpoint. We like to call this process 'the power of realistic thinking' when working with our patients.

E is the *evaluation* part of using the disputing thoughts to challenge the negative automatic thoughts. In this part, you assess how well your disputing thoughts are working to challenge your negative automatic thoughts and replace them with coping thoughts.

Table 13-1 takes you through two examples to show you how the ABC model operates.

Table 13-1	The ABC Model in Action	
	Scenario 1	*Scenario 2*
Activating event	You experience a mild increase in your heart rate and feel uncomfortable and jittery	You experience back or neck pain
Belief	I'm having a heart attack!	Something is seriously wrong with my spine. My spine is weak and fragile. Nobody really understands my pain.
Consequent emotions	Fear, anxiety, panic	Hopelessness, helplessness, anxiety, depression, anger
Resulting behaviour use	Call doctor or go to casualty	Slow, robotic movements; social isolation; irritability; of pain medication

In Scenario 1, you interpret your symptoms as a heart attack. Subsequent emotions and behaviour follow from this belief. Given the same activating event, an alternative belief may be 'I have just drunk four cups of coffee and I'm on a caffeine high.' With this explanation, your emotions and resulting behaviour are entirely different – even though the situation prompting the beliefs is exactly the same.

In Scenario 2, your pain triggers a number of negative automatic thoughts that are likely to make you feel worse. Negative emotions and other behaviours then follow from these negative thoughts. Alternative coping beliefs are 'My spine is a strong structure', 'I'm finding ways to manage this increase in back or neck pain', and 'I can choose to not allow the pain to control my life.' Again, you can analyse the same situation using different thoughts. Using coping thoughts results in more positive emotions and less pain.

Your beliefs – not the situation itself – cause your emotional responses and behaviour.

Using the three- and five-column techniques

The examples in Table 13-1 illustrate how your thoughts and beliefs influence your emotions and behaviour. But how can you use this information to help with your back or neck pain? You use the *three-* and *five-column techniques* to change your negative automatic thoughts to realistic, coping, and nurturing thoughts.

A *three-column worksheet* uses the ABC parts of the ABCDE model. Filling out the three columns on the worksheet enables you to run through your automatic negative thoughts in slow motion. Figure 13-1 shows an example of a three-column worksheet.

Activating Event	**B**eliefs	**C**onsequent Emotions
Sitting at work. Supervisor gave me too much to do. I'm noticing worse pain in my back as well as my neck.	There is something seriously wrong with my back.	Fear
	My spine is weak and fragile.	
	If I move the wrong way, I'll do myself in.	
	I'll never lead a normal life.	Helplessness
	I can't cope with this pain.	
	There is nothing I can do about this pain.	Hopelessness
	My back pain is all their fault.	Anger and Entitlement
	My boss doesn't understand my pain.	
	My boss expects too much from me.	
	I should be better by now.	Guilt
	I should never have let myself get injured in the first place.	
	This pain is ruining my family.	

Figure 13-1:
Example of a three-column worksheet.

What is stress?

Stress is defined as a mental or physical demand made upon your body. Your body responds to stress by increasing your blood pressure, heart rate, and breathing rate, tensing your muscles, and reducing blood flow to your head, stomach, skin, hands, and feet.

When you're tense, your body produces stress hormones to give you an energy burst. If you're in danger, these hormones help your body perform at maximum efficiency for survival by reducing gut function and diverting blood flow. But when these hormones are released inappropriately over a long time, they damage your body. Think of running your car's engine beyond its design capabilities: Fine for a quick getaway, but you blow up the engine if you do it too much.

Some studies suggest that stress causes up to 85 per cent of all medical problems. This fact doesn't mean that physical problems are all in your head, but instead emphasises how prolonged stress causes physical changes in your body that result in various medical conditions. Stress-related problems include headaches, back and neck pain, sleep problems, digestive disorders, and high blood pressure. Stress can worsen almost any medical problem and make surgical procedures more difficult at every stage – before, during, and after. As with medical procedures, the more stress you have, the less likely you are to prosper.

At first, you may have difficulty fleshing out your beliefs (column B) or automatic negative thoughts (column C) about a situation. Automatic negative thoughts often contain words such as *should*, *ought*, *must*, *never*, and *always*, for example 'I should be able to handle this pain better', 'I *ought* to be better by now', or 'I *must* be a terrible person with this pain.'

Often, identifying your emotional reactions first, and then working backward to identify your negative automatic thoughts and beliefs, can be easier.

After you become adept at identifying the ABC components of stress and pain, try expanding the three columns to the *five-column technique*: Simply add to your worksheet the columns for disputing thoughts and evaluation, as in Figure 13-2.

Your disputing thoughts (in column D) are constructed to attack and counter directly the negative automatic thoughts you wrote in column B. Use the evaluation column (column E) to record how your disputing thoughts affect your original negative thoughts, emotions, and overall stress.

Activating Event	Beliefs	Consequent Emotions	Disputing Thoughts	Evaluation
Sitting at work. Supervisor gave me too much to do.	There is something seriously wrong with my back.	Fear	Hurt does not equal harm. This pain does not mean injury.	Much less fear
I'm noticing worse pain in my back as well as my neck.	My spine is weak and fragile.		The spine is a strong structure.	
	If I move the wrong way, I'll do myself in.		I am not at risk for injury.	
	I'll never lead a normal life.	Helplessness	No one can predict the future.	More feeling of control
	I can't cope with this pain.		I'm learning ways to cope. I've made it through before.	
	There is nothing I can do about this pain.	Hopelessness	There are things I can do. They are . . .	Somewhat better
	My back pain is all their fault.	Anger and Entitlement	Blaming does not help me get better.	Mild decrease in anger
	My boss doesn't understand my pain.		My boss acts that way to everyone.	
	My boss expects too much from me.		I can get a lot done if I work steady and pace myself.	
	I should be better by now.	Guilt	I am trying to get better and working hard at it.	Guilt improved
	I should never have let myself get injured in the first place.		It was not my fault.	
	This pain is ruining my family.		There are things I can do to lead a quality of life regardless of the pain.	

Figure 13-2: Expansion of the three-column worksheet to five columns.

Recognising the Relaxation Response: More than Just Relaxing

Distinguishing between the 'relaxation response' and simply 'relaxing' is important. When we discuss relaxation training, our patients often ask us if they can simply do something they enjoy, such as listening to music or sitting out in the garden. Although these types of activities are certainly 'relaxing' they don't elicit the 'relaxation response'.

Practise makes perfect

Just like discovering any new skill, you need to practise the relaxation exercises we feature in this chapter in order for them to be effective. The following guidelines can help you establish a regular regime and get the most out of each session.

✔ **Practise once or twice a day.** Practising at least once a day is necessary in order to elicit the relaxation response. Initially, your relaxation sessions may take some time. As you practise regularly, you may find that the amount of time required to elicit the relaxation response decreases.

✔ **Find a quiet place to relax.** Practise your exercises in a place where you aren't going to be disturbed or distracted. Turn off your phone and try using a fan or air conditioner to block out noise as you practise.

✔ **Give a five-minute warning.** Give yourself and other family members a five-minute warning before you begin your exercises. This helps you and your family take care of loose ends before you practise your relaxation techniques.

✔ **Practise at regular times each day.** Setting up regular practise times increases the likelihood of you completing your relaxation exercises. Choose a time when you're most likely to complete the exercises. Don't practise when you're so tired that you're likely to fall asleep, such as just after a big meal or just before you go to bed.

✔ **Assume a comfortable position.** You may be comfortable lying flat on your back, with your legs extended and your arms comfortably at your sides. Depending on your pain, you may want to flex your knees or support them with a pillow. If this position causes

you pain, try completing your relaxation exercises while sitting or standing.

✔ **Loosen your clothing.** Loosen any tight clothing and take off things such as your shoes, belt, watch, glasses, and jewellery. The objective is to be as comfortable as possible as you practise the exercises.

✔ **Set aside your worries.** Try writing down all the things on your mind and then physically put the paper to one side before practising. You can focus better on the relaxation exercise if other concerns are documented for your attention after you finish your relaxation exercise.

✔ **Assume a passive attitude.** You need to *allow the relaxation response to happen.* Don't *try* to relax or control your body. Don't judge your performance. Focusing on your breathing is all you need to do: Relaxation occurs on its own.

The *relaxation response* involves a number of physical changes, including a decrease in your heart rate, respiration rate, blood pressure, muscle tension, metabolism, and oxygen consumption.

You can achieve the relaxation response only by regularly practising relaxation techniques. After you begin to elicit the relaxation response, you may notice feeling more relaxed in other areas of your life, even when you're not directly practising relaxation techniques. Achieving the relaxation response

✔ Reduces generalised anxiety.

✔ Prevents stress from building up over time.

✔ Increases your energy levels and productivity.

✔ Improves your concentration, memory, and ability to focus.

✔ Induces deeper, more restorative sleep and reduces insomnia and fatigue.

✔ Increases your awareness of your emotional state and feelings. (Being 'stressed out' tends to make you unaware of your feelings.)

You can use a variety of techniques and exercises to bring about the relaxation response, including breathing techniques, cue-controlled relaxation, imagery, biofeedback, and hypnosis. The following sections cover these techniques in greater detail.

Trying Different Types of Breathing

You may find it strange that we're discussing how to breathe properly. Breathing is essential for life, and most of us assume we know how to do it properly. In reality, very few people actually breathe in the healthiest way.

In our experience, breathing exercises are the easiest way to elicit the relaxation response. The exercises we describe in this section are straightforward and require minimal body movement.

You have two basic ways of breathing:

✔ **Chest breathing**, or shallow breathing, occurs when you expand your chest with each breath in, raise your shoulders, and tuck in your abdomen. The breaths tend to be shallow and short and may be irregular and rapid. Chest breathing tends to cause excessive tension in your neck and shoulders.

Chest breathing is often associated with high anxiety states in which you hold your breath and experience hyperventilation, shortness of breath, constricted breathing, or a feeling that you're going to pass out. You're more prone to chest breathing when under stress, which in turn decreases your ability to cope with that stress.

✔ **Abdominal breathing**, or diaphragmatic breathing, is how newborn infants breathe. Adults also breathe abdominally when they sleep. This is a very relaxed form of breathing and utilises oxygen better than chest breathing.

Unfortunately, most of us are chest breathers. However, developing your diaphragmatic breathing technique is a key component to eliciting the relaxation response.

Breathing awareness

Before you begin your breathing exercises, follow these steps to discover how you usually breathe:

1. **Lie down on your back in a comfortable place.**

   You may want to raise your knees, because this position can help reduce pain (see Figure 13-3). If you find lying on your back uncomfortable, try sitting in a chair.

2. **Close your eyes and place one hand on your breastbone and the other hand over your belly button.**

3. **Without trying to change the way you usually breathe, become aware of the part of your body that moves as you inhale and exhale.**

   The hand on your breastbone monitors chest breathing, and the hand over your belly button monitors abdominal breathing.

4. **Pay attention to which hand rises when you inhale – the one on your abdomen or the one on your chest?**

   If your abdomen moves up and down with each breath, you're breathing diaphragmatically. If your chest moves up and down with each breath, you may be more of a chest breather.

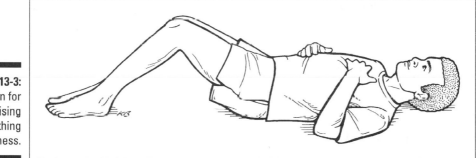

Figure 13-3:
Position for
practising
breathing
awareness.

Diaphragmatic or abdominal breathing

The following exercise helps you develop your abdominal breathing skills. Practise this exercise until you can breathe abdominally for five to ten minutes.

1. **Lie down in a comfortable position on your back, with your legs straight and slightly apart.**

   Allow your toes to point comfortably outwards and your arms to rest at your sides without touching your body. Place your palms up and close your eyes.

2. **Focus your attention on your breathing and place your hand on the spot that seems to rise and fall the most as you inhale and exhale.**

   Notice the position of your hand: It may be on your chest or abdomen, or somewhere in-between.

3. **Gently place both of your hands or a book on your abdomen and again focus on your breathing.**

Pay attention to how your abdomen rises as you inhale and falls as you exhale. Try to make your hands (or the book) rise and fall as you inhale and exhale.

Breathe through your nose during this exercise. You may need to blow your nose before doing your breathing exercises.

If you have difficulty breathing into your abdomen, press your hand down on your abdomen as you exhale and allow your abdomen to push your hand back up as you inhale deeply. The pressure from your hand helps you become more aware of the action of your abdomen during breathing.

4. **Take a few minutes and let your chest follow the movement of your abdomen.**

Notice whether your chest moves in harmony with your abdomen or whether it appears rigid. Continue to focus on making your abdomen move up and down as you breathe and allow your chest to follow your abdomen's motion naturally.

If you have difficulty breathing abdominally, try lying on your front, with your head resting on your folded hands. Take deep abdominal breaths so that you can feel your abdomen pushing against the floor as you breathe.

5. **As you practise abdominal breathing for five or ten minutes, scan your body for tension.**

Start at the top of your head and mentally scan your body down to your toes, searching for any tension. Tension hotspots that you may feel as you scan your body include your neck, shoulders, and back. If you find any tension, try and relax that part of your body more and more as you continue the breathing exercise.

Relaxed breathing

After you master abdominal breathing, try the following relaxed breathing exercise to begin to elicit the relaxation response:

1. **Lie down on your back.**

Bend your knees and move your feet about 20 centimetres apart with your toes turned slightly outwards. This position helps you straighten your spine and keeps you comfortable. You may be more comfortable if you place a pillow under your knees for extra support.

2. **Mentally scan your body for any tension, as we discuss in the preceding section.**

   You may notice tension as feelings of tightness or aching in a particular part of your body. If you notice any tension, make a mental note of it, for example, 'My shoulders and back feel a little tight'. You can rescan your body after the relaxed breathing exercise to see whether these tense spots have loosened up.

3. **Place one hand on your abdomen and one hand on your chest.**

4. **Inhale slowly and deeply through your nose into your abdomen, so that your hand rises.**

   Your chest should move only a little and should follow your abdomen.

   When you feel at ease with Step 4, move on to the deep breathing cycle, beginning with Step 5.

5. **Inhale through your nose while smiling slightly.**

6. **Exhale through your mouth, gently blowing the air out of your lungs and making a whooshing sound.**

7. **Take long slow deep breaths that raise and lower your abdomen.**

   Focus on the sound and feeling of breathing as you become more and more relaxed.

   Continue the relaxed breathing pattern for five or ten minutes at a time, once or twice a day. After doing this exercise daily for a week, try extending your relaxed breathing exercise period to 15 or 20 minutes.

8. **At the end of each relaxed breathing session, take time to scan your body for tension.**

   Compare the tension you feel at the conclusion of the exercise with that you felt at the beginning of the exercise. This gives you some idea as to how the relaxed breathing exercise is working. The more you practise, the better the exercise works.

As you become more proficient at relaxed breathing, you can practise at any time during the day in addition to your regularly scheduled sessions.

Considering Cue-controlled Relaxation

Cue-controlled relaxation is an effective technique you can use in conjunction with relaxed breathing or alone. In cue-controlled relaxation, you use a cue to signal the relaxation response. Although the cue can be anything, most people use a word that you say quietly to yourself, such as *relax*, *breathe*, or *one*; a phrase, such as *I am calm* or *My back and neck are relaxed*; or a line from a prayer.

Before trying cue-controlled relaxation, you need to have a basic mastery of relaxed breathing and eliciting the relaxation response. (See the section 'Trying Different Types of Breathing' for more information.) Practise relaxed breathing for at least a week before beginning cue-controlled relaxation.

To begin using cue-controlled relaxation:

1. **Choose a verbal cue.**

2. **Condition yourself to the cue.**

   Conditioning yourself to the cue means saying the cue (for example, the word 'relax') or seeing the cue (a spot) to cause your body to almost automatically relax. For conditioning to occur, you need to associate the cue with the relaxation response, much like thinking about food makes you salivate. Whenever you practise the relaxed breathing exercise, use the last several deep breaths at the end of your sessions for cue-controlled relaxation. If you choose a word cue such as 'relax', stretch out the sound of the word while you exhale and say 'reee-laax'. With practice, simply saying 'relax' to yourself in any situation can help you relax.

You can use cue-controlled relaxation in many situations where engaging in relaxed breathing is difficult or impossible or when you need to slow things down and decrease your pain or anxiety. For example, try using cue-controlled relaxation in the following situations:

- ✔ **To signal the relaxation response in any situation:** Use your cue to help you stay calm and relaxed, especially when you can't practise relaxed breathing.

- ✔ **To stop negative thoughts:** Cue-controlled relaxation is a powerful technique for stopping or disrupting negative and unproductive thinking. If you find yourself carried away by anxiety, distress, or negative thinking, use your cue to disrupt or stop these thoughts and redirect your thinking towards positive, coping statements.

- ✔ **To prepare yourself for an uncomfortable medical procedure:** Cue-controlled relaxation is an excellent way to prepare yourself for any medical procedure, particularly those related to your back or neck pain such as a nerve-block injection or to help you stay still during an MRI.

- ✔ **To manage an acute flare up of your back or neck pain:** Use your cue as soon as you experience increased pain to help you get through these episodes.

Cue-controlled relaxation is a very useful skill that you can call upon in a variety of situations. As with any skill, you need to take time to practise. The cue works for you only if you practise and give it a chance to become associated with your relaxation response.

Using Imagery Techniques

Imagery or *visualisation* – for example, picturing a pleasant situation or scene – is an excellent technique that can help you manage your back or neck pain successfully. In this section, we use the terms *imagery* and *visualisation* interchangeably.

Imagery is nothing magical. You engage in imagery every day: When you daydream or dream during sleep, you engage in imagery. Imagery is also used in athletic activities. You may imagine in your mind's eye the golf ball landing on the green before you hit the shot, or the football going into the goal before you take the free kick.

Day-to-day life offers ample evidence of the truth of this phenomenon. Think about what happens when you watch a scary film. During the film, your heartbeat increases, your palms become sweaty, and your breathing accelerates. These very real physical reactions occur in response to something that isn't real. The film simply activates your imagination and your brain responds, not knowing whether the monster is in the room or on the screen.

The attraction of distraction

Distraction is defined as causing a person to turn away from an original focus or attention. Clinical experience and research show that distraction can be a powerful technique for managing stressful medical procedures and controlling pain. Distraction techniques involve helping your mind to focus on something other than the stressful event. You can use the imagery exercises we discuss in this section as a method of distraction because they keep your mind busy and turn your attention away from your pain.

You may have already discovered your own distraction techniques for coping with stressful medical situations One study interviewed patients after they had undergone uncomfortable, stressful medical procedures, such as an MRI for back pain, and found that patients employed distraction methods such as counting the holes in ceiling tiles, repeating words or poems, singing and humming, engaging in conversation, and whistling.

Other distraction techniques include staring at a stationary object or a spot on the wall (a focal point), tapping the rhythm to a song with your finger or foot, and listening to music.

The benefits of imagery

Your natural ability to imagine can be used for many beneficial health purposes:

✔ **To enhance physical healing.** Many imagery exercises are designed to activate your body's natural ability to heal itself. Some imagery techniques include thinking about images such as white blood cells attacking germs or injured tissues receiving valuable nutrients from increased blood flow. Imagery exercises can be especially useful in healing a back or neck injury and in managing your pain. For instance, imagine the muscle around your spine as a bunch of tied up knots that you slowly loosen and undo as a way to decrease muscle tension.

✔ **To relieve your pain.** Imagery can help you remove yourself from the experience of pain. Using imagery techniques, you can mentally put yourself in another place to decrease your perception of pain and discomfort.

✔ **To improve your sleep.** Sleep disturbances are not uncommon if you have back or neck pain. Imagery can promote sleep. Often, sleeping imagery involves *passive* techniques in which you imagine your body feeling the physical sensation of relaxing, for example feeling warm and heavy.

✔ **To promote muscle relaxation.** This type of imagery involves activities such as imagining your muscles unwinding like the knots in a twisted rope, seeing a ball of tension in your body dissipate each time you exhale, or feeling your muscles become smoother and looser.

✔ **To distract you from a stressful medical procedure.** Imagery can be effective when you undergo an unpleasant or painful medical procedure. Imagery in which you guide your imagination through a sequence of events such as walking on the beach or down a forest path is particularly effective for this purpose.

Practising imagery

As you develop your imagery exercises, you need to decide which imagery approach works best for you. Remember that imagery is a natural process and you're always in complete control. Think of imagery as if you're a film director – you can project whatever image you want on to your mental screen.

As you develop your own imagery exercises, keep in mind the following:

✔ **Pre-record your imagery exercise.** Pre-recording your imagery exercise on audiotape can help your regular practice and make the experience as robust as possible.

Your first task is to write out your imagery script, including the places where you pause. Consider recording the breathing techniques from earlier in this chapter before the imagery exercise. Then record the script on to a tape. When making an audiotape of this type, read through the script very slowly and pause often. Speak in a calm, comforting, and steady voice. Let your voice flow in a smooth and somewhat monotonous manner, without whispering.

✓ **Use a familiar image.** Our clinical experience and much of the research suggest that patients who use images that are familiar to them have more success with this technique. Generally, people have an easier time conjuring up all aspects of the image when they've actually experienced the image. So, choose something like a beach or forest that you have visited and that has pleasant associations for you. This way, you have a better experience with all the elements of the image.

Images developed from your own memories and experiences don't have to contain the entire memory. You can draw from bits and pieces of different memories in order to form a complete image.

✓ **Use all five of your senses in developing the image.** For instance, if you imagine a beach scene, notice the view of the sea and the beach, the smell of the water, the sounds of the seagulls and the waves crashing, the taste of the sea air, and the feel of your bare feet walking on the warm sand.

✓ **Use an image pleasing to you.** The old adage 'One person's feast is another person's poison' applies to imagery, which is a personal, individualised experience. Make sure that your imagery is pleasing to you.

✓ **Sneak up on the image.** Sometimes focusing immediately on an entire image at one time can be difficult. Research suggests that 'sneaking up on the image' can be a helpful technique: Construct the image slowly in order to avoid becoming frustrated in creating the scene. For example, if using a forest scene as your image, begin by imagining that you're at home preparing to go to the forest or on your way to the forest. Imagine driving to the end of the road, getting out of the car, and walking slowly into the beautiful mountain scene that is your final goal image. Using this technique helps ensure that the imagery is relaxing and that you adopt an attitude of letting it happen, rather than trying too hard.

✓ **Use one image at a time.** Trying to maintain several images at once is stressful and usually fails to accomplish the goal of imagery.

✓ **Precede the imagery with a relaxation exercise.** Using a relaxation exercise, such as those we discuss throughout this chapter, can greatly improve your use of imagery.

✓ **Make your relaxation and imagery session 10–20 minutes long.** Depending on your pain, you may have trouble sitting or lying down for more than 10–20 minutes, but aim for a minimum of 10 minutes. A session shorter than 10 minutes doesn't give you enough time to relax and develop the image. Also, trying to do imagery quickly can cause you to rush and defeat the purpose. As you practise, you may want to go longer than 20 minutes, which is fine.

✔ **Practise the image.** The ability to create a mental image using all five senses may be difficult at first but does improve with practise. If your images aren't vivid initially, don't worry. As you practise, more details come into focus, and you feel more and more as if you're actually in the image.

✔ **Develop a technique to end your image gradually rather than stopping it abruptly.** One of the most common side effects of using imagery is feeling slightly drowsy afterwards. Using a technique to end the image can help avoid this problem. One of the most common methods is to count silently from one to five. Then, on the last count, inhale deeply, open your eyes, and say to yourself 'I feel alert and relaxed.'

Trying some standard imagery exercises

Have a go with the following imagery example, or develop a more individualised, personal example. In the example here, the series of dots represent places where you pause in order to develop a slow pace to the exercise:

✔ **Passive muscle relaxation:** When you feel ready, allow your eyes to close slowly . . . Take in a full, deep breath through your nose, allowing your lungs to fill completely. Let the air go in all the way, breathing down into the bottom of your lungs. Notice the cool sensation in your nose as the air rushes in . . . Breathe out through your mouth while slightly pursing your lips . . . Notice that the air you exhale is warm and moist . . . Release all the air in your lungs as you exhale completely . . . Repeat this cycle slowly, several times.

Allow yourself to relax more and more fully. Begin to focus your attention on your fingers and hands . . . Notice the sensations coming from that part of your body . . . Imagine what it would feel like for your hands and fingers to become more and more relaxed . . . Let go of any excess tension you may feel in your fingers or hands.

As you continue to relax and breath peacefully, slowly move your mental attention to the sensations coming from your forearms and upper arms . . . As your fingers and hands continue to relax, allow that feeling of relaxation to move into your forearms and upper arms . . . You may notice your hands or arms feeling warm or heavy as they relax. Or you may notice them feeling cool and light . . . Simply focus on what the relaxation response feels like for you. As your arms continue to relax with every breath, allow the feeling of relaxation to move into your head, neck, and shoulders . . . Let your forehead relax completely . . . Allow the muscles around your eyes to relax . . . As you relax the muscles of your jaw, you may notice that your lips separate slightly . . . Allow your shoulders to relax completely . . .

When you're ready, focus your attention on the sensations coming from your stomach and back. Imagine what it would be like for all the muscles in your stomach and back to unwind and loosen up completely . . . Act as if you're inhaling relaxation and exhaling tension with every breath . . . As you continue to enjoy this feeling of relaxation, imagine the pleasurable sensation moving into your upper legs . . . Notice how the relaxation spreads throughout all the muscles of your legs and feet . . . Again, you may notice your entire body becoming heavier and heavier, or lighter and lighter. You may also notice a tingling sensation as part of the relaxation response. These normal feelings are part of relaxing . . . Simply focus on what the relaxation sensation feels like for you. . . .

The preceding passive muscle relaxation exercise can lead to other imagery scenes such as a beach scene or a pain reduction scene. The following are parts of these types of images that you can expand upon:

- **The beach scene:** Imagine that the time is about five o'clock in the afternoon on a midsummer's day. You're walking along a shady path that opens up to a beautiful and expansive beach. As you walk from the path onto the sandy beach, you notice that the beach is virtually deserted. The deep and golden sun hasn't yet begun to set, but is very low on the horizon. The sand is warm and comfortable on your toes, and you notice the taste and smell of the salt in the sea air. You settle deeply into the comfortable sand dune as you enjoy the sun's reflection off the water.

- **Breathing out pain:** Imagine your breath goes to that part of your body where you experience pain or discomfort. Each time you breathe in, imagine the healthy air flowing to that area of your pain and discomfort. Each breath brings a sensation of health and comfort. Each time you breathe out the air, notice the area of pain and discomfort becoming smaller and smaller. As you breathe out, you exhale discomfort and pain. Continue to breathe in the relaxation and breathe out the pain.

Humour, health, and back and neck pain

'A cheerful heart is good medicine.' —Proverbs 17:22

Laughter and humour are fun, but they can also improve your mood, reduce emotional tension, exercise your cardiovascular system, and promote social interactions. As well as these more obvious benefits, a physiological basis may well exist for the conclusion that laughter is good medicine. Studies demonstrate that laughter can provide such health benefits as decreasing pain sensitivity, improving sleep, and boosting your immune system.

Try using your humour for health as follows:

- Expose yourself to humour through films, jokes, books, and television.

- Keep a humour journal in which you record funny thoughts and experiences.

- Tell a joke and be able to laugh at yourself.

- Look for the funny side of a stressful situation. Sometimes laughing about a stressful situation is the only control you can exert — so you may as well have fun with it!

- Spend time with happy, optimistic people.

Beginning Biofeedback Training

Biofeedback training measures a physical process such as your heart rate or brain waves and reports the information back to you so that you can develop the ability to influence that physical state consciously. Biofeedback can measure a variety of things, including the following:

- ✔ Skin temperature, which is influenced by blood flow beneath your skin.
- ✔ Galvanic skin response (GSR), which is the electrical action of your skin due to the activity of your sweat glands.
- ✔ Muscle tension, which can be measured by electromyography (EMG).
- ✔ Heart rate, which is easy to assess.
- ✔ Brain wave activity, which can be measured and recorded by the electroencaphalogram (EEG).

For instance, if increased muscle tension contributes to your pain, monitoring tension and thus becoming able to decrease it can help you relieve your pain. If anxiety is a problem, monitoring your heart rate and galvanic skin response can help you decrease your anxiety. Monitoring any of these systems can also help you achieve a general state of relaxation.

Biofeedback training is a painless, non-invasive procedure. The practitioner places electrodes on your skin to monitor the muscle to be retrained, as shown in Figure 13-4. This muscle may be an area of soreness, spasm, or suspected muscle imbalance. The computer connected to the electrodes measures the amount of electrical activity present in the muscle, related to tension. You can see the amount of 'tension' on the monitor and gradually become able to decrease it. Your brain 'learns' how to decrease the muscle tension simply by having the feedback available.

We recommend a short trial of biofeedback of say 5–15 sessions when muscle tension appears to be part of your back or neck pain or you're anxious about your symptoms.

The essential feature of biofeedback training is discovering how to relax without needing the equipment. This aim is most often achieved through relaxation training and using relaxation tapes at home.

Beware of practitioners abusing biofeedback training, requiring you to attend too many sessions and keeping you dependent on the biofeedback machines. Some research indicates that the biofeedback machine itself may not be necessary and that you can achieve the same results through relaxation training. Even so, we do find a significant effect in the patient being able to 'see' the changes occur as the process takes place.

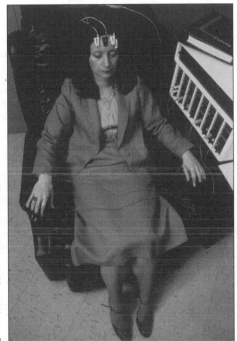

Figure 13-4:
Not a
bizarre
scientific
experiment,
but a patient
undergoing
biofeedback
training.

Take a look at www.netdoctor.co.uk and www.ability.org.uk/
biofeedback.html to find out more about biofeedback.

Homing In on Hypnosis

Hypnosis is a natural state of focused concentration that makes relaxing and
controlling your mind and body easier. Hypnosis is a sleep-like condition in
which the subject goes into a trance but responds to the suggestions of the
hypnotist. Since Franz Anton Mesmer, considered to be the father of hypnosis, first discovered this fascinating technique more than 200 years ago, hypnosis has seen cycles of acceptance and rejection. Currently, hypnosis is
used widely to treat many psychological and medical conditions, including
back and neck pain. Hypnosis can also be a useful tool to help you manage
stressful medical procedures such as nerve blocks and MRI scans and as a
preparation for spinal surgery.

Make sure that a licensed psychologist or doctor, or qualified hypnotist performs any hypnosis for your spinal problems. You may find that you pick up
the hypnotic skills from your professional so that you can use self-hypnosis
to duplicate the effects.

The hypnotic process involves the following:

- ✔ **Relaxation:** In hypnosis, relaxation is induced. This usually includes relaxed breathing similar to the breathing we describe in the exercises earlier in this chapter.

- ✔ **Imagery:** Relaxation exercises and healing imagery help to deepen your level of hypnosis. Often, the hypnotist uses imagery to deepen your level of relaxation, such as asking you to imagine going down some steps, an escalator, or a lift.

- ✔ **Suggestion:** The hypnotist presents *hypnotic suggestions* that address your specific needs, for example to control your back or neck pain or to reduce your stress during medical procedures. Suggestions may include the following:

  - Breathing comfortably and deeply makes you stronger.

  - You feel calm and relaxed. You have nothing to worry about. You can set your troubles aside until you heal.

  - You will sleep soundly.

You can make specific suggestions a part of your pain-management programme by repeating the suggestions during your relaxed breathing and imagery exercises. If you choose to give yourself hypnotic suggestions, a process known as *self-hypnosis*, make sure that the suggestions are realistic, for example: 'When I tell myself to relax, I will notice less pain', 'I will feel more and more confident throughout the day', or 'Each time I hear the phone ring, I will feel more relaxed.'

You may notice that an overlap exists between the relaxation response, cue-controlled relaxation, and hypnosis. These techniques have similar features that you can combine into an effective pain-management programme.

We know of no reported cases of harm resulting from hypnosis. If you're interested in using hypnosis as part of managing your back or neck pain, we recommend you seek professional help from a qualified health care professional. Your professional should have special training in hypnosis dealing with medical problems, such as back or neck pain or managing stressful medical procedures.

The World Health Organisation suggests that hypnosis is not to be performed on certain people, such as people with psychosis or other psychiatric conditions.

For more information about hypnosis, check out the resources listed in Appendix B, and see *Hypnotherapy For Dummies* by Mike Bryant and Peter Mabbutt (Wiley).

Seven hypno-myths

Widespread misconceptions about hypnosis, particularly perpetuated by stories in the media and films, have limited its use in clinical and professional settings. Here are seven of the most common misconceptions:

✔ **Hypnosis is a state of deep sleep or unconsciousness.** Hypnosis is actually a state of relaxed attention in which you can hear, speak, move around, and think independently. Your brain waves in a hypnotic state are similar to those when you're awake. Reflexes that are absent when you sleep, such as your knee reflex, are present when you're hypnotised.

✔ **You must be gullible, weak-willed, or passive to be hypnotised.** Actually, the opposite is true. Because their powers of concentration are better, individuals most responsive to hypnosis tend to be more intelligent, creative, and strong-willed. The primary factor in benefiting from hypnosis is a strong motivation to participate.

✔ **Hypnosis allows someone else to control your mind.** This belief is probably not only the biggest misconception about hypnosis but also the one that keeps people from pursuing and benefiting from hypnosis. You can't be hypnotised against your will. Once hypnotised, you can't be forced to do something you find objectionable.

✔ **You may not be able to come out of a trance.** Actually, becoming hypnotised is more difficult than coming out of hypnosis. If left alone and hypnotised, you become alert and awaken naturally in a short period of time.

✔ **Under hypnosis, you may give away secrets.** When hypnotised, you're aware of everything that happens, both during and after hypnosis, unless you want to accept and follow some specific suggestions for amnesia. Your hypnosis professional can't force you to express secrets that you're unwilling to divulge.

✔ **You probably can't be hypnotised.** Although some people are more responsive than others, almost everyone can achieve some level of hypnosis and can benefit from it with practise. Challenges to hypnosis include trying too hard, fears or misconceptions about hypnosis, and unconscious desires to hang on to troublesome symptoms. A licensed hypnosis professional can help you overcome these stumbling blocks.

✔ **Hypnosis is a quick, easy cure-all.** This misconception is due to extravagant and inaccurate claims regarding hypnosis. Such claims are detrimental and result in a loss of credibility for the overall practice.

Part IV
Rehabilitation

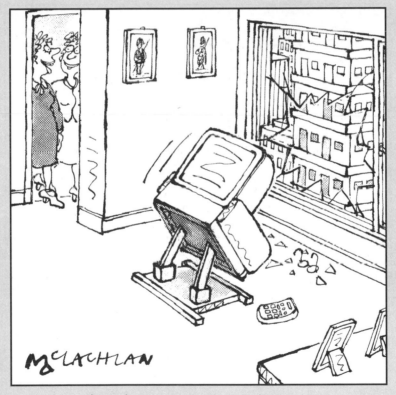

"Let's hope that new luxury
recliner we bought for Grandad
has helped his back pain"

In this part . . .

*E*ven if you never pinpoint the exact cause of your back or neck pain, your doctor (or other healthcare professional) will devise a treatment programme for you. By following your doctor's recommendations, you can manage your pain and return to all your normal activities. However, carrying out the treatment plan is up to you.

This part is hands-on. We tell you what things your doctor is likely to ask you to do, we help you design a solid back and neck exercise programme, and we give you tip after tip of things that you can do on your own. We also throw in a few useful back and neck products that can help alleviate pain, or at least make you more comfortable.

Chapter 14

The Importance of Posture

*W*hen we talk about 'posture', you may remember being told as a child to 'Stand up straight!' or 'Don't slouch!' Good posture keeps your back and neck healthy, but a healthy spine involves more than standing to attention.

Posture can be divided into two categories:

✔ **Static posture** is the position of your body when you're stationary. Standing and sitting are examples of static posture.

✔ **Dynamic posture** is the position of your body as it moves. Walking, bending, and lifting are examples of dynamic posture.

Understanding the look and feel of healthy static and dynamic postures can help you prevent back and neck pain, or better manage your back and neck pain when it does occur. In this chapter, we help you identify when your posture is unhealthy and show you how to improve your posture.

Sizing Up Static Postures

Even though you're not moving, static postures can place unnecessary pressure on your spine if you assume an unhealthy position. Most people spend a great deal of time standing, sitting, and lying down during a typical day. Understanding how to be in these positions comfortably may play an important role in your back and neck health.

Standing up for yourself

As an individual, you have a unique standing position that is efficient, comfortable, and healthy for your back and neck. Your ideal standing posture supports your body in a balanced, upright alignment with minimal use of muscle energy and no perception of strain.

Examining your standing position

A good way to assess your current standing posture is to stand sideways before a full-length mirror.

If you have two mirrors available, place the mirrors at an angle so that you can look straight ahead into one and get a side view of yourself from the other. Using two mirrors avoids you having to turn your neck to the side to observe your posture.

As you look in the mirror, assume a posture that is an exaggeration of your normal standing posture. For instance, if you tend to slump your shoulders, slump them more. Or, if your abdomen tends to stick out, push it out more. Although not your everyday posture, this exaggerated posture can help you identify problems as you go through the following list. Assume your exaggerated posture and ask yourself these questions:

- ✔ **Are my knees locked or bent?** Ideally your knees are relatively straight, but not entirely locked.

- ✔ **What's going on with my lower back, pelvis, and abdomen?** Ideally, your waistline, and thus your pelvis, is fairly level, with your lower back having only a mild curve and your abdomen tucked in. This position is called a *pelvic tilt*, which we describe in Chapter 15. We give you more tips on how to achieve this position in the section 'Adopting healthy standing habits'.

- ✔ **Are my shoulders slumped over?** Ideally, your shoulders are in a straight line with your torso and not rounded forwards and slumped over.

- ✔ **Are my head and neck tilted forwards from my shoulders?** Ideally your head is fairly centred over the top of your chest and in a level position, and your neck is fairly straight, with a slight forward curve.

As you check yourself out in the mirror, you may notice some unhealthy aspects of your standing position. See whether your stance has any of the following features:

✔ **The military stance:** Many children assume this stance when told to 'Stand up straight!' In this position, you stand as straight, tall, and rigid as you can (see the left-hand example in Figure 14-1). The military stance may look good, but isn't healthy for your back and neck. This stance can cause your lower back to curve more than it should (causing your abdomen to stick out) and your head to tip backwards over your neck, which strains the ligaments and muscles of your upper back.

✔ **Slumped posture:** In this posture, your head is tilted forwards, your shoulders are slumped forwards and down, and your abdomen sticks out, increasing the curve of your lower back (see the right-hand example in Figure 14-1). Slumped posture may irritate and put excessive strain on structures in your lower back. The tilted head and extra curve of your spine can also cause neck pain.

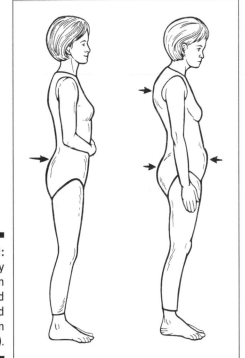

Figure 14-1: The military stance (on the left) and the slumped posture (on the right).

Adopting healthy standing habits

After assessing your posture using the mirror technique we describe earlier in this section, try to adopt a healthy standing posture, as shown in Figure 14-2.

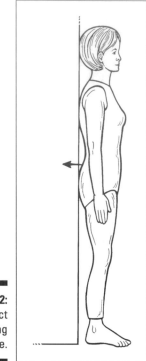

Figure 14-2:
Correct
standing
posture.

A healthy standing position may feel uncomfortable at first, especially if you've been 'practising' an unhealthy standing posture for 30 years or more. Rest assured that you can develop a better standing posture and doing so can help you feel better.

To practise a healthy standing position, stand against a wall with your heels approximately 6 centimetres away from the wall. (Standing slightly away from the wall allows room for your buttocks.) Do a standing pelvic tilt: Move the small of your back towards the wall by tilting your pelvis. Keep your knees slightly bent and make sure not to lock them in a straight position.

The *pelvic tilt* is a healthy standing posture. Practising the pelvic tilt exercise while lying down, as demonstrated in Chapter 15, can help strengthen your abdominal muscles, which help you maintain a healthy posture while standing.

The following guidelines can help you develop a healthy standing posture:

✔ **Use a footrest when standing for an extended length of time.** Most people stand with both feet on the ground, as the 'incorrect standing posture' in Figure 14-3 shows. The right-hand part of Figure 14-3 shows how placing one foot on a low stool or stack of books gives you a healthier standing posture. Alternate your feet every once in a while. This position reduces the curve in your lower back and decreases the strain on the facet joints (which we describe in Chapter 2) in your lower spine.

✔ **Avoid bending or leaning over when standing for an extended period of time.** For instance, bending over a sink as you work in the kitchen places quite a bit of strain on your lower back. When you need to maintain a bent or leaning posture for a long time, bend your knees slightly to absorb some of the strain on your lower back.

✔ **Reduce the time you spend wearing high heels, as these shoes increase the curve of your lower back, possibly placing more strain on it.**

✔ **Place commonly used household items at eye level to stop the need for repetitive bending.**

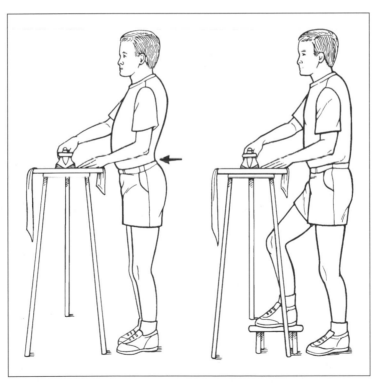

Figure 14-3:
Incorrect (without the footstool) and correct (with the footstool) posture for long periods on your feet.

> ✔ **Try to move about and alternate your position frequently (about every 20 minutes) when standing for a long period of time.** Change positions to keep your muscles and spine relaxed. Repetition of any activity over a prolonged period of time can cause your muscles to become fatigued and eventually may cause pain.

As you become more aware of your unhealthy habits, try to substitute them with healthy habits, which may decrease your back and neck pain.

Sitting casually

Research suggests that sitting in the same position for an extended time is more stressful on your back than standing, lying down, and even, in some cases, lifting. Sitting stresses your back because your muscles have to work harder to keep you upright and stable. When your back isn't well supported as you sit, your muscles tire quickly. You then tend to slouch to give your muscles a break. Slouching causes your centre of gravity to shift forwards and your pelvis to rotate backwards, which puts your lower spine in an unnatural position. This unnatural position means that the discs of your lumbar spine bear the weight of your entire upper body unevenly. Studies show that pressure between discs increases with sitting. Although some well-designed chairs can decrease stress on your spine, many people sit on the edge of their chair out of habit, which defeats the point of the chair's design.

Assessing your sitting posture

By assessing your own sitting posture, you can determine whether you sit in an unhealthy way and what to do to change your posture. First, sit in a chair and exaggerate your normal, comfortable sitting posture. To help you do this, try moving yourself away from the backrest and allowing your entire upper body to 'let go' and relax. You can imagine a side view of your posture in this position, or you can look at yourself in a mirror as described in the section 'Examining your standing position'.

In the exaggerated posture, assess yourself for the following characteristics:

> ✔ **Slumped posture:** If your sitting posture is slumped, your lower back tends to be rounded out, your chest depressed inwards, your upper back rounded forwards, and your neck arched backwards in order to keep your head level. Your head probably feels like it is projecting out in front of your chest rather than being balanced above your torso.
>
> Slumped sitting greatly increases the pressure on your lower back. In this position, the middle and upper joints of your neck tend to be crammed together because of the increased backward arching. The muscles of

your neck and shoulders are also overworked in this position. After sitting in this position for an extended period of time, you may find straightening up into a standing position quite difficult.

✓ **Tense sitting:** In this type of sitting, you sustain a certain level of tension in your muscles because your back is unsupported, you're in a stressful situation, or simply through general tension. People who engage in tense sitting are often not even aware that their bodies are tense until a practitioner monitors their muscle tension through biofeedback (which we describe in Chapter 13).

Tense sitting can occur in conjunction with unhealthy or healthy posture. For example, you may maintain a healthy posture but have almost all the muscles in your body in a state of low-level tension. Becoming aware of muscle tension and practising relaxation (which we talk about in Chapter 13) can help reduce this muscle tension.

✓ **Sitting too long:** Your body isn't designed to be in a sitting position for an extended period of time with no movement. Even when you sit correctly, try to get up and move your body regularly. Sitting for long periods of time puts undue strain on the structures of your back, including the muscles.

✓ **Crossing your legs:** For short periods of time, crossing your legs is comfortable and allows your muscles to relax. Staying in this position for an extended period of time, however, causes some of the same problems as sitting for too long. Crossing your legs as you sit in a chair that doesn't provide support causes you to hold a slumped or tense sitting posture.

First, become aware of whether you tend to cross one particular leg over the other consistently. If you do, try to switch legs regularly to help cancel out the imbalance in your posture. Then pay attention to keeping your legs uncrossed when you can.

Sitting pretty (and healthily)

The first rule of healthy sitting is to become aware of whether you experience any of the unhealthy patterns we describe in the preceding section. The following healthy sitting guidelines can help you sit more comfortably and reduce the stress on your lower back:

✓ **Position your pelvis:** Healthy sitting involves paying attention to the position of your pelvis, because your pelvis affects the position of your lower back and your entire upper body. To position your pelvis properly, move your tail bone back as far as possible in the chair with your upper body tilting forwards (imagine tucking your buttocks into the back of the chair). After you tuck your pelvis into the back of the chair, bring your body into the upright position. This move repositions your pelvis into a healthy posture. You may need to adjust this position slightly (for example, rolling your pelvis slightly forwards or backwards) until it feels good for you. Figure 14-4 shows the entire process.

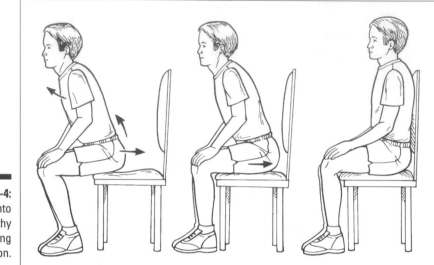

Figure 14-4:
Getting into
a healthy
sitting
position.

✔ **Keep your pelvis, chest, and head aligned:** After you become familiar
with a healthy sitting position, change your position frequently and keep
stressful forces on your lower back to a minimum. The primary goal is to
keep your pelvis, chest, and head aligned whether you're sitting back,
up, or forwards. Thus, as your upper torso leans backwards, your lower
body needs to tilt upwards to maintain the proper posture or angle
between your upper and lower body. We show a healthy sitting posture
at a desk (including angles for the elbows and knees) in Figure 14-5.

  • If you're sitting with your pelvis well back in the chair (and your
    upper body slightly backwards), you may want to place a small
    footstool (often designed with a slant to fit your feet) or telephone
    book under your feet (see Figure 14-5). Using a footstool helps
    raise your knees slightly above hip level, which puts your pelvis in
    a healthy position.

  • If you're sitting on the edge of a chair, try to keep your knees lower
    than your hips, move your legs wider apart than normally (two to
    three feet), and position one foot forwards and the other foot far-
    ther back on the floor.

✔ **Use a good chair:** Getting a chair designed for healthy sitting is very
important, especially if you sit for extended periods of time on a regular
basis, such as at work. The more you sit, the more your body takes on
the shape of the particular chair you use (although changing positions
frequently does help). The sidebar 'Buying a chair' talks about how to
shop for a good chair.

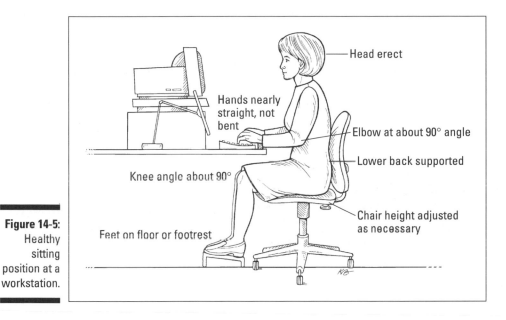

Figure 14-5:
Healthy
sitting
position at a
workstation.

Labels in figure:
Head erect
Hands nearly straight, not bent
Elbow at about 90° angle
Lower back supported
Chair height adjusted as necessary
Knee angle about 90°
Feet on floor or footrest

✔ **Use a proper support in an unsupported chair:** If you use a chair that doesn't provide proper support, you can take steps to improve your sitting position. First, if the chair doesn't provide support for your lower back, put a rolled-up towel, small cushion, or commercially available lumbar-support pillow behind the small of your back to help keep the natural curve of your lower back when sitting. Second, if you tend to sink down in the chair, as often happens in soft couches, put a folded towel or even a book under your buttocks to fill in the part of the seat you sink into.

✔ **Take breaks and move around:** One of the best ways to keep your back and neck healthy while sitting is to take frequent breaks and move around. Making yourself take breaks may be quite a challenge, especially if you're engrossed in a task and don't realise that you've been sitting in the same position for two or three hours. If you're prone to sitting too long, try setting a timer for about every 30 minutes to remind you to get up and take a break. In your break, try simple activities such as walking around or doing some of the stretching exercises we describe in Chapter 15.

Lying down on the job – and anywhere else

One of the first areas to assess for healthy lying down is your mattress. If your bed is too soft, your spine relies on your muscles and ligaments to keep its natural shape, which may increase your muscle tension and the stress on your spine.

Buying a chair

When you go shopping for a back- and neck-friendly chair, you may find the number of choices overwhelming. Gathering information about the various chairs is important. Choosing the best chair for you depends upon factors such as your body shape and the type of work you need to do as you sit in the chair. Ask a physiotherapist or a well-trained salesperson at some of the stores that specialise in these products (Appendix B lists these specialist shops).

Try to follow these general guidelines when buying a chair:

✔ Ensure that the chair supports and maintains your spine in its natural shape as you sit. The curve in the small of your back needs to be neither excessive nor reduced but maintained in its natural form. When you're not using a chair at a desk, try a chair that tilts back slightly and has a footrest to support your feet.

✔ Check that the height of a desk chair is easily adjustable. When the seat of your chair is too high, the curve of your lower back increases to an unhealthy position, your feet almost dangle, and the muscles of your upper and lower back are strained. Most good chairs have a hydraulic mechanism for changing height.

✔ Make sure that the chair provides lumbar support for your lower back. Most high-quality (unfortunately, another word for *expensive*) office chairs provide this essential support. When the muscles of your lower back aren't supported properly, they contract. This low-level muscle contraction, when sustained for many hours, causes muscle fatigue and spasm, which may lead to back pain.

✔ Avoid a chair that you 'sink into' deeply. A really soft chair causes the muscles in your lower back to tense as they attempt to provide your spine with the support that the chair lacks.

✔ Choose a chair with a curved front edge, as a sharp edge that puts undue pressure on your upper legs can decrease blood flow to your thighs and lower legs.

✔ Select a chair that transfers the majority of your weight to your buttocks rather than your thighs as you sit. Some chairs are so straight-backed that they push your upper body forwards, putting pressure on your thighs.

✔ Choose a chair with armrests, if possible. Armrests can help decrease the tension and fatigue on your neck and shoulders, and also help you stabilise the chair when making the transition from sitting to standing and vice versa.

Simply putting a piece of plywood between the bed springs and a soft mattress is *not* a reasonable solution to sleeping on a soft mattress. You simply create a situation in which your soft mattress presses into the hard surface of the board – which causes the mattress to wear out sooner. Using a board under a mattress can help, however, if you have a good mattress on a sagging metal frame that provides inadequate support for the mattress. The sidebar 'Choosing a mattress' covers how to shop for a mattress that is both comfortable and kind to your back and neck.

Even if you have a decent mattress, lying down in an unhealthy position can still create back or neck problems. A great deal of advice is available on proper sleeping positions, but the research isn't clear on whether different sleeping positions affect your back or neck pain. Sleeping positions may be an individual thing: For you they may be important, but for other people they may not matter.

The important thing is for you to be comfortable when lying down. Try some of the following tips, remembering that your overall comfort is the most important thing as you sleep:

- **Solving the 'sleeping on your front' problem:** Lying on your front increases the curve of your lower back. If you can't give up sleeping on your tummy, try to straighten out your spine by placing a pillow or towel under your pelvis.

- **Solving the 'sleeping flat on your back' problem:** Lying flat on your back with your legs outstretched increases the curve in your lower back and may cause stress to that area. If you prefer to sleep on your back, support your hips by bending your knees and placing a pillow underneath them. This solution places your lower back in a natural, comfortable position.

- **Using the foetal position:** In this position, you lie on your side, with both hips and knees bent equally. Placing a small pillow between your knees may make you even more comfortable. Also, you can put a small pillow under your head and neck to fill the space between your head and shoulders.

- **Being aware of the sofa:** Think of your sofa as a small soft bed. Lying down on the sofa, whether to sleep, watch TV, or read, may cause the same stresses as lying on a soft bed. Instead, try lying on your back on the floor with your knees bent over some pillows or a chair. You can place a small pillow under your neck to support your head.

Dealing with Dynamic Postures

Dynamic postures are the positions your body takes when in motion. Movement requires your muscles, ligaments, and bones to work together in a co-ordinated fashion. Proper dynamic posture involves the most efficient way of moving and using the posture most likely to prevent injury to your spine.

Paying attention to proper dynamic posture is a little more difficult than appreciating static posture because you may not have as much time to plan ahead. In the following sections we review healthy dynamic postures.

Choosing a mattress

You have many options when it comes to buying a mattress. Mattresses and bed springs are designed to work together to provide support for your body. The following bed tips can help you make a good choice:

✔ A well-made mattress and bed spring set lasts between 7 and 15 years, depending on the quality and how you take care of the bed.

✔ Proper bed maintenance includes turning the mattress end to end and upside down every month for the first few months so the mattress adjusts evenly to your body weight. After that time, turn the mattress every couple of months. Of course, if you have back or neck pain, get help turning your mattress and make sure that you use proper lifting techniques (see 'Bending and lifting in a healthy manner' later in this chapter).

✔ A third of your life is spent in bed, so invest your money wisely. Ensure that you spend at least five or ten minutes seeing how it feels in the showroom. Some shops offer a mattress exchange service to allow you to try the mattress for 30 days at home.

✔ Most mattresses use a spring coil construction, but they vary greatly in terms of the number and thickness of the coil springs. Finding a bed that is comfortable for you is a highly individual choice. Just like Goldilocks, you want a mattress and box spring set that is neither too firm nor too soft but that provides enough support to keep your back in its natural curves.

Ask for specific information about different bed and mattress features at a speciality mattress store. You can even discuss this information with your physiotherapist or other health care professional.

Walking tall

Walking is your most basic form of transportation, as well as being good exercise.

Checking out the way you walk

We suggest you evaluate your walking posture for unhealthy habits. A good way to assess your walking is to watch yourself, sideways on, walking, in a mirror or even in the reflection of a shop window. Try to exaggerate your movements, so if you tend to walk with your head forwards or your abdomen pushed out, direct your head up more or push your tummy out a bit more. If you walk fairly loosely and casually, loosen up even more. If you walk in a fast, rigid manner, exaggerate those qualities. Understanding the unhealthy patterns of walking you engage in can help you correct those patterns and adapt to using the healthy walking patterns we describe later in this section. The following unhealthy walking patterns may put more stress and strain on your lower back:

✔ **Abdomen-out walking:** Increasing the forward arch of your lower back, along with stretching out your lower stomach, causes your pelvis to tilt forward as you walk. This alignment can aggravate lower back pain. In this unhealthy walking posture, you tend to walk with your abdomen leading far out in front of the rest of your body.

✔ **Head-forward walking:** Looking down at the ground directly in front of you while you walk generally causes this pattern. You also put your chest in a depressed position, which causes stress on your neck, shoulders, and lower back. Head-forward walking results in shallow breathing and overall endurance.

✔ **Loose walking:** A tendency to be wobbly and engage in extraneous movements of the joints of your legs, arms, neck, and back characterises this pattern. You may be prone to this type of walking if you have a tendency toward joint instability and muscle weakness.

✔ **Stiff walking:** This pattern is the opposite of loose walking and can be due to being tense and uptight, having a fear of falling or re-injury, or being concerned about making your back or neck pain worse. People who walk stiffly look like they have a corset or brace from their neck to their lower back (or, in more severe cases, from their head to their toes). This type of walking looks very robotic. Stiff walking causes your muscles to work too hard as they try to prevent any motion from occurring around your neck and back. This muscle overactivity tends to pull all the joints of your body together in a state of total body contraction. Stiff walking causes you to tire rapidly due to the amount of energy you expend to maintain rigidity. Stiff walking actually increases the probability of injury and pain flare ups in your back.

✔ **Heel-pounding walking:** A heavy heel- or foot-strike each time you take a step characterises this walking pattern, as if you're pounding out a beat as you walk. This type of walking sends shock waves from your foot to your leg and up to your pelvic and spinal joints. The shock waves create extra stress throughout these body parts. This type of walking is usually developed through habit and is more exaggerated when you're in a hurry, emotionally upset, barefoot, or wearing hard or stiletto heels.

✔ **Stress walking:** Taking fast, choppy steps, with your upper body held forwards and your head down, characterises this pattern of walking. Similar to the heel-pounding walk, stress walking transmits shock waves from your lower body to your pelvis and spine. Stress walking involves total body muscle tension, especially around areas of pain such as your lower back or neck. You may stress-walk as a matter of habit and find that it gets worse when you're under emotional pressure.

Becoming a healthy walker

Before attempting healthy walking, identify whether you exhibit any of the unhealthy patterns we describe in the preceding list, to help you focus on healthy walking techniques. Here are some tips for healthy walking:

✔ **Make your pelvis level.** Keep your hips and lower back in a stable position as you walk. This tip involves doing a slight pelvic tilt (which we explain in Chapter 15) as you walk. Imagine a straight line coming directly out of the centre of your bellybutton as you walk. Generally, that line points at a downward angle. In order to get a slight pelvic tilt, imagine shifting the line up slightly. Doing this slight shift while you walk results in a tilt that brings your pelvis to a more level position and makes walking easier on your spine.

✔ **Release tension as you walk.** Use breathing techniques (check out Chapter 13 for help with these) as you walk to keep the muscles of your body, including your back, in a relaxed state. Each time you slowly exhale while you walk, think about releasing any tightness that is holding your body rigid. This technique can help prevent stiff walking, stress walking, and heel-pounding.

✔ **Keep your head light.** Thinking in terms of keeping your head and neck light on your shoulders as you walk can help you walk better. Allow your head and neck to relax and simply 'ride', centred and at ease, on top of your shoulders. This technique helps decrease any tension you may be carrying in your shoulders or neck.

✔ **Use a soft landing.** As you walk, think about your legs moving smoothly and your feet landing softly as they touch the ground with each step. Try to reduce the amount of pounding and the shock waves generated throughout your body. Focus on landing each foot more quietly, softly, and smoothly. You can walk smoothly but still walk as quickly as you need to. The shoes you wear can help you walk more smoothly and decrease heel-pounding: Especially good shoes are trainers with a well-fitting heel, room for the front of your foot, proper support, and excellent cushioning.

✔ **Walk smoothly.** As you walk, allow your head and trunk to be relatively upright in order to maintain a healthy posture and improve breathing. Limit any extra movement of your hips, and keep your head from tipping forward, backward, or off to either side. Try to minimise any twisting between your various body parts, such as your upper and lower body. Visualise your face, shoulders, chest, and hips being in a relatively stable position and facing forward while you walk. Healthy walking involves a smooth motion of the muscles of your legs and feet.

Looking at lifting and bending

Lifting and bending are commonly associated with the onset of spinal pain. When you use unhealthy bending and lifting techniques, you place a significant amount of pressure and strain on your spine each time. Repeated bending and lifting can cause back and neck pain even if the things you lift are very light. Following healthy lifting and bending techniques is one of the most effective ways to reduce undue stress on your spine.

Buying a pair of shoes

The type of shoes you wear can affect how your back and neck feel when you stand and walk. Your shoes determine how your lower body interacts with the ground in two ways: positioning and transmission of shock waves. No matter what shoes you wear, whether athletic or dressy, when buying a pair of shoes pay attention to the following basics of healthy footwear:

✔ The *heel counter* is the part of the shoe that surrounds your heel and needs to be stable enough to hold your heel upright while you stand and walk. Make sure that the heel counter is made of reinforced and durable material. When the heel counter is weak, your heel can move inwards or outwards, increasing strain on your legs and your lower back.

✔ The *heel* of the shoe is the platform under the bones of your heel. The heel needs to be well-padded to absorb shock and elevated slightly above the ball of your foot. Ensure that the width of the heel is equal to the width of the heel counter in order to help distribute the shock from walking. Hard and dense heels increase the amount of shock transmitted from your legs to your back. High heels can cause an unstable effect on the legs that may increase muscle tension in the lower back.

Beware of heels that have worn unevenly, because they can cause you to walk and stand unevenly.

✔ The shoe needs to have a reasonable amount of flexibility at the ball of the foot to provide a smooth motion while walking. When the sole of the shoe is too rigid, it doesn't 'give' when you try to bend it. A stiff sole not only is uncomfortable but also causes you to walk in an unnatural, unhealthy way. On the other hand, a sole that is too flexible and soft doesn't give your feet the proper support that they need (especially in the arches).

✔ The *insole* is the inside flat part of the shoe extending from the toes to the heel. The insole of your shoe needs to provide comfortable support to the heel and arch of your foot. Check inside one of your shoes, and you should see a contour that matches the shape of the bottom of your foot. A good insole has a build-up of material to support the arch. When this build-up is missing, your feet tend to fall inwards and flatten out, putting your lower body into a state of misalignment that increases pressure on your lower spine. A podiatrist can advise you on custom-made insoles.

✔ The *toe box* is the part of the shoe that surrounds your toes. The toe box needs to allow enough room for your toes to move around while providing adequate support on both sides of your foot. The side support must prevent your toes from moving excessively from side to side, but in no way cramp or squeeze your toes. Ensure that you don't feel the top of your toes hitting the roof of the toe box.

Identifying unhealthy bending and lifting

Like many people, you may just go up to the object you need to lift, bend over, grab it, and pick it up. You do so without thinking or planning ahead because, in most cases, you can get away with it and don't injure your back or neck – which shows the amazing strength of your spine. Unfortunately, the one time you don't get away with it, but instead sustain a back or neck injury, can be the start of an ongoing back or neck pain problem. The following safety tips, in addition to the others discussed in this chapter, can help you avoid injuring your back and neck.

Read through the following characteristics of unhealthy bending and lifting, and pick out those that you commonly engage in. Identifying your bad habits helps you to become aware of them and adapt to healthier techniques instead:

- **Standing with your feet too close together:** One of the most common unhealthy ways to bend and lift is with your feet too close together. When your feet are closer than shoulder-width apart, you have poor leverage, are unstable, and tend to round your back as you bend and lift.

- **Bending at the waist:** Another unhealthy way to move is to bend at your waist while keeping your knees and hips straight and arching your lower back forward. An example of this move is shown in Figure 14-6. Bending at the waist is probably the most common and stressful way to lift anything: And twisting at the same time makes things even worse.

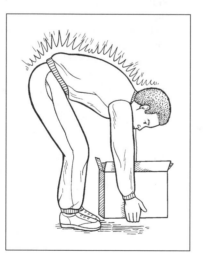

Figure 14-6: Incorrect lifting posture.

- **Lifting and carrying an unbalanced load:** Examples of this common, unhealthy manner of bending and lifting include carrying a heavy suitcase in one hand with nothing in your other hand or carrying a heavy bag on one shoulder.

- **Lifting objects that are too heavy for you:** Lifting, or trying to lift, something that is really too heavy for you places a strain on your back and neck. An example is trying to lift something in one big 'strained' move.

✔ **Lifting and bending repetitively:** This unhealthy move is a common cause of work injuries, where you repetitively bend and lift within a short period of time without taking breaks. If you get tired from repetitive bending and lifting, you probably have a poor technique, which increases your chances for injury.

✔ **Lifting objects at a distance from your body:** Another common mistake is attempting to lift an object away from your body. Lifting a 4.5-kilogram (10-pound) weight 35 centimetres (14 inches) from your body, rather than being close to it, is equivalent to lifting approximately 68 kilograms (150 pounds) as far as your spine is concerned. Lifting even a light object at a distance from your body puts a great deal more pressure on your spine than lifting close to your body.

Bending and lifting in a healthy manner

If you follow some healthy bending and lifting guidelines, you can reduce your chances of back or neck injury and help prevent future flare ups of pain. Most of these tips involve using common sense and not taking shortcuts:

✔ **Place your feet at the proper width apart.** When bending and lifting, ensure that your feet and knees are at least shoulder-width apart if side by side. If your feet are one in front of the other, they need to be in a wide step position. Positioning your feet in this manner helps you bend at the hips and keeps your back relatively straight and unstressed.

✔ **Use your legs when lifting.** When bending and lifting, bend your knees so that your legs take on most of the stress. Squat with your chest sticking out forwards and your buttocks protruding out backwards. This position helps keep your lower back straight and puts a minimal amount of pressure on your back (see Figure 14-7).

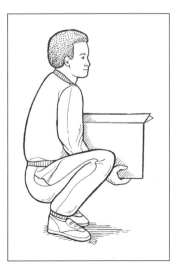

Figure 14-7:
Preparing to
lift properly.

✔ **Keep the weight of the object close to you as you lift.** As you lift and carry something, keep the object as close to your body as possible. When lifting a heavy object from a full squat, keep your elbows and forearms in contact with the insides of your thighs. This technique helps you to be more stable and transfers more weight off your spine and on to your legs – a proper squat lift.

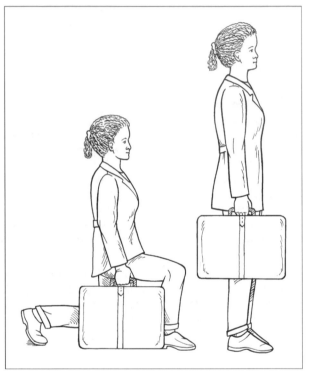

Figure 14-8:
The half-kneeling lifting technique.

Another good lifting technique is the half-kneeling lift, as shown in Figure 14-8. This technique is good for lifting large items such as suitcases and bags of shopping. Go down into a half-kneeling position and then push up with both legs to a standing position. Keep your upper torso straight as you lift. If the object is heavy and doesn't have handles, use the half-kneeling position to roll the object onto your raised thigh. From this position, you can hold the item close to your chest and push up with your legs from the half-kneeling position to a standing position. Ensure that you keep your back straight throughout this manoeuvre.

✔ **Carry a balanced load.** Try to balance your load on both sides of your body. Rather than carrying a heavy bag of shopping on one side, divide it into two lighter bags that you can carry on either side. If that isn't an option, switch sides frequently so that you balance the stress on your body across both sides. When you have a very heavy load, avoid carrying it altogether. Instead, use a cart to push the load or ask somebody for help. Remember: Using the correct technique may take a little more time, but helping to prevent a back or neck injury is well worth a few extra minutes.

✔ **Avoid lifting objects above waist level.** If possible, don't lift things above your waist and certainly not above your shoulders. Both of these postures increase the curve of your lower back, placing unnecessary strain on the muscles, ligaments, and joints in that area. You are much more vulnerable to a lower back injury when you lift an object above waist or shoulder level.

✔ **Keep your arms straight.** Try to keep your arms as straight as possible when lifting an object while using your legs. Make sure that your arms are straight down, not straight out. With your arms straight down, your leg muscles (which are much stronger) do most of the work.

✔ **Remember that lowering objects is also stressful.** Lowering an object may seem easier than lifting it, but lowering can also cause stress and strain on your lower back. Many people injure their back or neck when losing control of a heavy item while lowering it, and then grabbing to prevent the item from hitting the floor.

✔ **Lift at a moderate speed.** Lifting an object at a moderate speed, using a smooth motion, neither too fast nor too slowly, is best. Lifting too fast can cause you to use unsafe techniques and lose control of the object. On the other hand, lifting too slowly can also make you unstable and increase the time that your lower back is under stress.

✔ **Beware of odd-shaped objects.** The most difficult type of object to lift is one that is irregularly shaped, heavy, and with no handles. If you need to lift such an object, get help from someone else or find a way to avoid lifting the object altogether.

✔ **Plan ahead.** Before lifting anything, the most important safety technique is to plan ahead. Unfortunately, this step is most often overlooked. Planning ahead helps ensure that you use proper lifting techniques or avoid lifting an object that is more likely to cause a back or neck injury altogether.

✔ **Avoid twisting when lifting.** One of the worst things you can do is twist as you lift an object. Twisting and lifting places a great deal of pressure on the structures of your lower back and can result in a disc herniation or other injury (see Chapter 3). Instead, pick up the object using one of the healthy techniques we describe earlier in this section and then turn your entire body to face where you want to put the object. This technique avoids putting any twisting motion on your back.

✔ **Push rather than pull.** In most cases, pushing a heavy object is easier than pulling it. Pushing a heavy object along the floor places less stress and strain on your lower back. In so doing try to bend mainly at your hips and knees, and try to keep your spine as straight as possible.

✔ **Pay attention to maximum lifting guidelines.** Generally, the maximum lifting load for women is 14–18 kilograms (30–35 pounds) and for men about 25–30 kilograms (50–60 pounds). When you need to lift an object much heavier than these guidelines, consider getting help or using some other technique to avoid lifting, such as a cart or dolly. Or simply unpack the box a bit if it's overloaded!

✔ **Ask someone to help you lift.** Two people are better than one when it comes to lifting heavier objects. Make sure that the weight of the object is distributed as evenly as possible. Break up the journey by moving the object a short way, placing it down and having a rest, and then moving it another short distance.

Chapter 15

Exercising Your Way to a Healthy Back and Neck

A regular exercise programme helps keep the muscles of your neck, back, and abdomen strong and flexible, giving your back support and decreasing the chances of an attack of spinal pain. Even if you've never had significant spinal pain, exercises can help prevent future injury. Exercising can also ease chronic back and neck pain.

This chapter presents a comprehensive back and neck exercise programme, which we suggest you combine with some type of aerobic conditioning, such as walking, bicycling, or swimming. A good way to ensure that you get both types of exercise is to do your back and neck exercise programme on one day, followed by aerobic conditioning the next day, and so on.

General aerobic conditioning is important not only for your back and neck but also to improve muscle tone, to relieve stress, to improve your sleep, and for lots of other benefits that we discuss in Chapter 8.

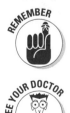

Consult your GP or specialist before starting any type of exercise programme, including a back or neck conditioning programme. Talking with your doctor first is especially important if you haven't exercised for some time or you have risk factors that your doctor needs to monitor, such as heart disease or high blood pressure.

Exercise Tips

To make your exercise programme safe, beneficial, and effective, try to follow these tips when exercising:

- ✓ **Set aside time to exercise.** Plan ahead. Make sure that you are undisturbed during your exercise time. The exercise regimen in this chapter takes some 15–30 minutes to complete and is most beneficial when you do it three to five times a week.

  If you choose to exercise first thing in the morning, walk around a little bit after getting up before doing your exercises.

- ✓ **Exercise on a firm but comfortable surface and wear loose-fitting clothing.** Carpeting or an exercise mat provides a good exercise surface. Don't exercise on a very soft surface such as a bed or couch, as soft surfaces don't provide your body with adequate support.

- ✓ **Move slowly and smoothly.** Especially when you're just beginning an exercise programme, concentrate on making your movements easy and graceful. Take a brief rest between each exercise if you find that helps you complete the programme.

- ✓ **Go at your own pace.** When beginning an exercise, do the number of repetitions that cause you little or no discomfort. Increase your repetitions using the quota system that we discuss in Chapter 8. For example, start out with two or three repetitions of a particular exercise and add one repetition per week until you reach your goal.

  Make sure that at no point during your exercise programme do you feel that you're straining beyond your physical capabilities or to the point of significantly increasing your pain.

- ✓ **Make a public commitment.** Tell as many people as possible about your exercise programme. Making this commitment to exercising helps ensure that you follow through with this healthy idea.

- ✓ **Get an exercise buddy.** Set up a regular exercise time and regimen with a friend. This makes you accountable to someone else and therefore less likely to cancel or drop out of your exercise programme.

- ✓ **Focus on your breathing.** As you progress through your exercises, focus on healthy breathing, as we discuss in Chapter 13. Try to breathe evenly and deeply. Avoid holding your breath or taking shallow breaths.

  Inhaling slowly through your nose and exhaling slowly through your mouth is a good technique to ensure healthy breathing.

Exercise Warnings

Just as we offer some tips to enhance your exercise programme, we also have some specific warnings:

✔ **See your doctor if you experience numbness in the genital area, sexual problems, or muscle weakness in your legs.** If you experience any of these symptoms contact your doctor immediately. Refer to Chapter 6 for in-depth information on these and other warning signs. Of these, numbness in the genital area is absolutely critical. Proceed to your local A&E department immediately.

✔ **Don't start your exercise programme in the middle of an acute attack of pain.** Wait until your pain calms down before starting on the exercises, unless your doctor recommends otherwise. This waiting period may be anything between one day and three weeks after the onset of your pain.

✔ **Expect some soreness and discomfort after exercising.** If you haven't stretched or strengthened your muscles for some time, those muscles may be sore after you exercise. For this reason, start your exercise programme at a very low level such as two or three repetitions of each exercise. Your exercise programme is sure to be more enjoyable and less painful if you do it regularly. Soreness is normal in any individual and is temporary, it will probably come on over 24–72 hours after exercising and will reduce over the same period.

If at any time you experience a dramatic increase in pain, any of the warning signs discussed previously, or any new type of pain, see your GP. If you have difficulty doing the exercises due to an increase in your pain, stop that exercise for a few days and then return to it at a lower level of repetitions.

✔ **Don't bounce.** Bouncing is fine for Tigger in *Winnie-the-Pooh*, but it has no place in stretching exercises. Stretch using a gradual, smooth, slow motion. Don't stretch beyond what you find comfortable. Using a bouncy or jerky motion puts you at risk of muscle and ligament injury.

Your Exercise Programme

Our exercise programme is excellent for strengthening and stretching the muscles of your lower back and abdominal area. The exercise regimen takes 15–30 minutes, depending on the number of repetitions of each exercise you do. Begin the programme slowly and gradually work up to more repetitions as you become stronger.

The following sections outline a general back and neck conditioning programme. Your practitioner may recommend a slightly different programme, depending on your symptoms. You follow the first part of the exercise programme as you lie on your back. Then you move to lie on your front and then take up a position on your hands and knees. You do the final exercises while standing.

The zigzag line in the figures shows the parts of the body that each exercise focuses on.

Exercise 1: Pelvic tilt

This exercise stretches your abdominal and back muscles and increases the flexibility of your pelvis and hips (see Figure 15-1).

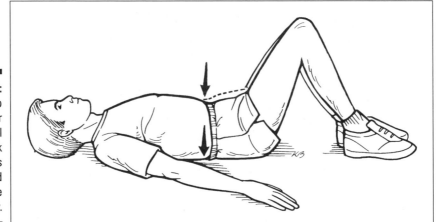

Figure 15-1:
Pelvic tilt to stretch your abdominal and back muscles and increase flexibility.

1. **Lie on your back with your knees bent, your feet flat on the floor, and your arms at your sides.** Your feet should be about hip-width apart, and your knees slightly closer together than your feet.

2. **Flatten the small of your back against the floor.**

   This causes your hips to tilt upwards.

3. Hold this position for a few seconds and then relax.

Breathe in as you do the pelvic tilt, and breathe out as you relax.

Begin with two or three repetitions if you can, and gradually work your way up to between five and ten repetitions.

Exercise 2: Single leg pull

This exercise stretches the muscles of your hips, lower back, and buttocks (see Figure 15-2).

1. **Lie on your back with one leg bent, one foot flat on the floor, and your other leg extended straight out.**

2. **Use the arm on the same side to draw the bent knee to your chest in a continuous motion while keeping your lower back and other knee pressed against the floor.**

3. **Hold this position for a count of five seconds – (say 'One rhinoceros, two rhinoceros, three . . .'). Keep breathing normally.**

4. **Slowly lower your leg to the starting position.**

Repeat this movement two to five times with the same leg.

5. **Switch legs and repeat Steps 2–4.**

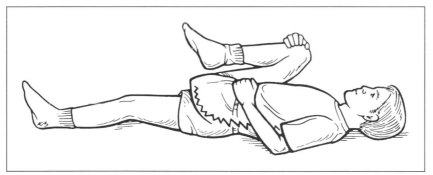

Figure 15-2:
Single leg
pull to
stretch your
hips, lower
back, and
buttocks.

Exercise 3: Double knee to chest

This exercise stretches the muscles of your hip area, buttocks, and lower back (see Figure 15-3).

1. **Lie on your back with your knees bent, your feet flat on the floor, and your arms at your sides.**

   Your knees should be far enough apart to be comfortable for you (usually fairly close together for this exercise).

2. **Raise both knees to your chest.**

   Use your arms to pull your knees gently to your chest.

3. **Hold for a count of five.**

4. **Lower your legs one at a time to the floor and rest briefly between each repetition.**

Begin with two or three repetitions and work your way up to 10–20 repetitions.

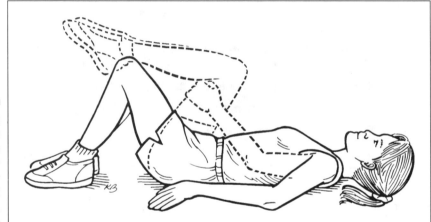

Figure 15-3: Double knee to chest to stretch your lower back and buttocks.

Exercise 4: Pelvic lift

This exercise strengthens the muscles of your buttocks (see Figure 15-4).

1. **Lie on your back with your knees bent, your feet flat on the floor at about shoulder width, and arms at your sides.**

2. **Raise your hips bit by bit, as shown in Figure 15-4.**

   Raise your hips without arching your back. Focus on not sticking out your abdomen to stop you arching your back. Try to keep a straight line from your shoulders to your knees.

3. **Hold for a count of five (follow the mantra we give in Exercise 2).**

4. **Slowly lower your hips to the starting position.**

Begin with two or three repetitions and gradually work up to five.

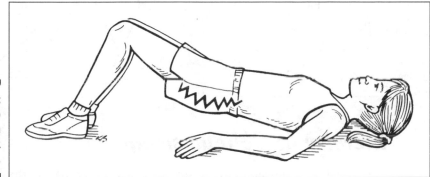

Figure 15-4:
Pelvic lift to
strengthen
your buttock
muscles.

Exercise 5: Partial sit-up

This sit-up strengthens your abdominal muscles (see Figure 15-5).

1. **Lie on your back with your knees bent, your feet flat on the floor, and your arms by your sides.**

2. **Cross your arms over your chest and, keeping your middle and lower back flat on the floor, raise your head and shoulders off the floor slightly, as shown in Figure 15-5.**

   Raise up only far enough to get your shoulder blades just off the floor. Don't worry if you can't go up too far at first.

3. **Hold this position for just a few seconds.**

   As you get stronger, you can work up to holding the position for five to ten seconds.

4. **Gently return your upper body to a relaxed position on the floor.**

Start out with two or three repetitions and gradually increase to between five and ten repetitions.

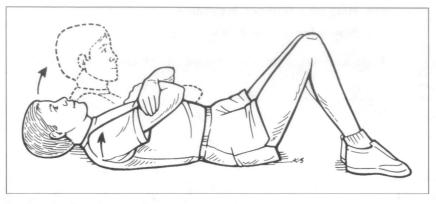

Figure 15-5:
Partial
sit-up to
strengthen
your
abdominal
muscles.

Exercise 6: Oblique sit-up

This variation of the sit-up works your *oblique muscles*, part of the abdominal wall that act like an elastic corset to support you and also play an important part in spinal movements.

1. **Lie on your back with your knees bent and your feet flat on the floor. Place your hands behind your neck.**

2. **Lift one side of your upper back off the ground and rotate your elbow toward your opposite knee (see Figure 15-6).**

   Move slowly and in a controlled manner. Don't use momentum from your arms to perform the move.

3. **Return to your original position.**

4. **Repeat this motion with your other arm leading the way.**

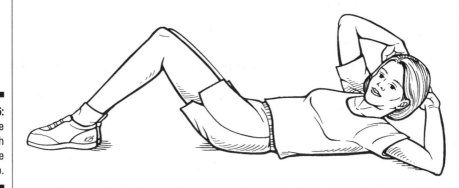

Figure 15-6:
Doing the
twist with
the oblique
sit-up.

Exercise 7: Hamstring stretch

This stretch works the backs of your thighs (see Figure 15-7).

1. **Lie on your back with one leg bent, one foot flat on the floor, and your other leg extended straight out.**

2. **Lift your straight leg (the one flat on the floor) upwards until you feel a slight stretch along the back of your leg.**

   Use your hands to grasp behind your knee and help raise and hold your leg, as in Figure 15-7. If you have difficulty reaching your knee with your hands, place a towel under your knee or thigh and pull up on that. Don't worry if you have a slight bend at the knee in the leg you're stretching – keeping it perfectly straight is a feat reserved for Olympic gymnasts.

3. **Hold the position for 30 seconds.**

4. **Slowly lower your leg down to the floor.**

5. **Switch legs and repeat Steps 2–4.**

Do two or three repetitions on each leg to begin with, and work your way up to five repetitions.

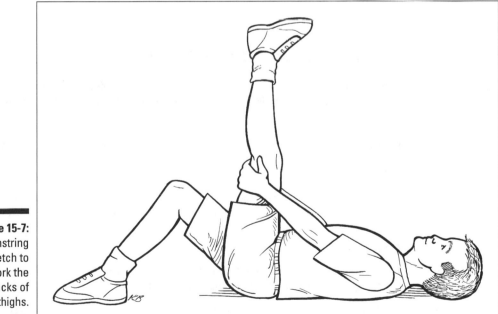

Figure 15-7:
Hamstring
stretch to
work the
backs of
your thighs.

Exercise 8: Gentle press-up

This exercise stretches the muscles of your abdominal area and provides some upper-body strengthening.

1. **Lie on your front with your feet slightly apart. Place your face near the floor or rest your forehead on the floor, and put your hands palm-down at face level, as shown in the first image in Figure 15-8.**

2. **Use your arms to push the top half of your body gradually to a resting position on your elbows, as in the second image in Figure 15-8.**

   You may feel tightness in your lower back or abdomen. Try to hold this position for 20 seconds or more if you feel comfortable.

3. **Push up with your arms, keeping your hands on the floor, as high as possible while keeping your hips and legs flat on the floor (see the third image in Figure 15-8).**

   Remember to keep your back relaxed.

4. **Hold the position for 20–30 seconds. Keep breathing normally.**

5. **Slowly lower yourself back to the floor.**

Initially do two or three repetitions, and work your way up to about five repetitions.

Exercise 9: Cat and camel

As the first image in Figure 15-9 shows, this exercise uses a new starting position. This exercise is designed to strengthen your back and abdominal muscles.

1. **Start on your hands and knees, with your weight distributed evenly and your neck parallel to the floor, as shown in the first image of Figure 15-9.**

2. **Arch your back upwards by tightening your abdominal and buttock muscles, letting your head drop slightly, as shown in the second image in Figure 15-9.**

3. **Hold for a count of five.**

4. **Let your back sag gently towards the floor while keeping your arms straight, as shown in the third image in Figure 15-9.**

   Keep your weight distributed evenly between your legs and arms.

5. **Hold for a count of five again.**

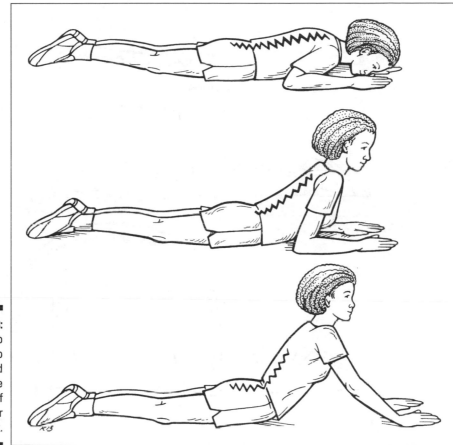

Figure 15-8:
Press-up
exercise to
stretch and
maintain the
curve of
your lower
back.

Do two or three repetitions initially and work your way up to about five repetitions. Be sure to make your movements slow and smooth.

Inhale through your nose as you arch your back and exhale through your mouth as you let your back sag.

Exercise 10: Arm reach

This exercise strengthens the muscles of your shoulders and upper back (see Figure 15-10).

1. **Start on your hands and knees, with your weight distributed evenly and your neck parallel to the floor.**

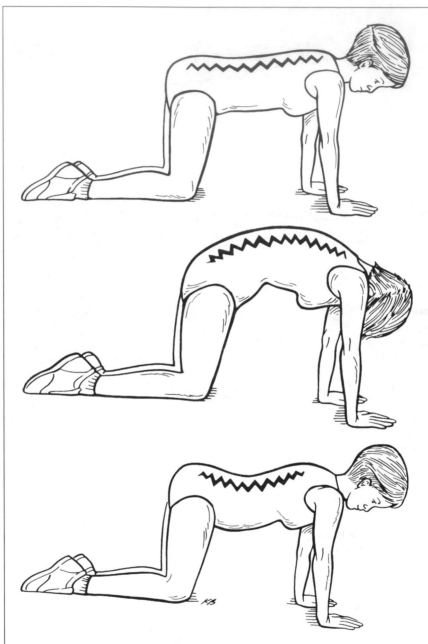

Figure 15-9:
Cat and
camel
exercise to
strengthen
your back
and
abdominal
muscles.

2. **Stretch one arm out in front of you, being careful not to raise your head.**

   Keep your weight distributed evenly between your knees and the one arm on the floor.

3. **Hold the arm reach for a count of five.**

4. **Return to the starting position.**

5. **Do five repetitions with the same arm.**

6. **Switch to your other arm and repeat Steps 2–5.**

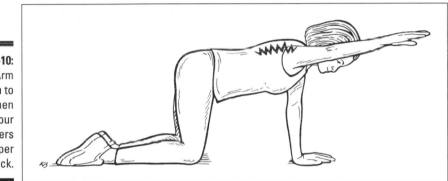

Figure 15-10:
Arm reach to strengthen your shoulders and upper back.

Exercise 11: Leg reach

This exercise is designed to strengthen the muscles of your buttocks (see Figure 15-11).

1. **Start on your hands and knees, with your weight distributed evenly and your neck parallel to the floor.**

2. **Slowly extend one leg straight out behind you and hold it parallel to the floor.**

   Your foot may be pointed or flexed – whichever is comfortable for you.

   As you extend your leg, don't let your back, head, or stomach sag. And make sure that no one is behind you when you do this!

3. **Hold the position for a count of five.**

   You may be able to hold this pose for only two or three seconds when you start out. This length of time is typical when first practising this exercise; your endurance improves as you gain strength and stability through practise.

4. **Return to the starting position and repeat this movement three to five times.**

5. **Switch legs and repeat Steps 2–4.**

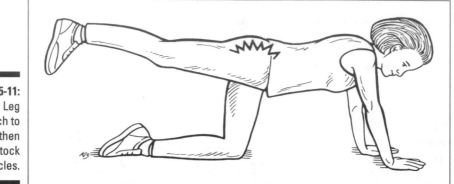

Figure 15-11:
Leg stretch to strengthen your buttock muscles.

Exercise 12: Alternate arm and leg reach

If you find this challenging exercise difficult initially, practise Exercises 10 and 11 for a few weeks before adding this one to your programme (see Figure 15-12).

1. **Start on your hands and knees, with your weight distributed evenly and your neck parallel to the floor.**

2. **Extend one leg backwards, parallel to the floor (as we describe for Exercise 11), and at the same time reach forwards with the opposite arm (as we describe for Exercise 10).**

   Try to make your leg, torso, head, and arm form a straight line parallel to the floor.

3. **Hold this position for a count of three.**

4. **Lower your leg and arm to the starting position.**

5. **Repeat the same movements with your other side.**

Work your way up to five repetitions of this exercise on each side.

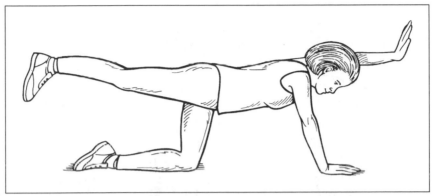

Figure 15-12:
Alternate arm and leg reach to help strengthen your shoulders, upper back, and buttocks.

Exercise 13: Wall slide

Although the name sounds like a new dance step, the wall slide is actually a valuable exercise that strengthens your back, hip, and leg muscles – as you can tell after doing it!

1. **Stand with your back against a wall and your feet shoulder-width apart, as shown in the first image in Figure 15-13.**

   Place your hands on your hips or let your arms hang at your sides, whichever is more comfortable. Keep your head level by focusing directly in front of you.

2. **Slide down the wall into a crouched position with your knees bent to about 90 degrees, as in the second image in Figure 15-13.**

   If you have trouble going down this far, slide down halfway.

3. **Hold this position for a count of five.**

4. **Slide smoothly up to your starting position.**

Initially, you may be able to complete only two or three repetitions of this exercise. Your goal is to complete five repetitions while holding the crouched position for one minute each time. Work up to this goal gradually.

Exercise 14: Side stretch

After completing Exercise 13, step away from the wall and remain standing. This side stretch exercise stretches the muscles in your back and sides (see Figure 15-14).

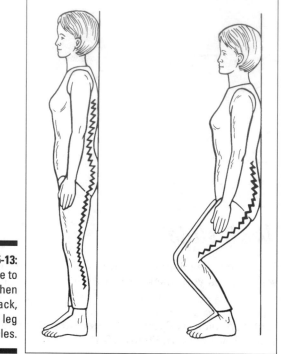

Figure 15-13:
Wall slide to strengthen your back, hip, and leg muscles.

1. **Stretch one arm over your head and bend your upper body to the opposite side in a fluid motion.**

   Put your other hand on your waist. Don't twist your body as you bend or lean forwards.

2. **Hold the stretch for a count of five.**

3. **Return to the starting position with your hands and arms at your sides.**

4. **Repeat this movement five or more times.**

5. **Switch to the other side and repeat Steps 1–4.**

Do this stretch with a flowing movement and avoid jerking.

Exercise 15: Back arch

The back arch stretches your shoulder, back, and hip muscles (see Figure 15-15).

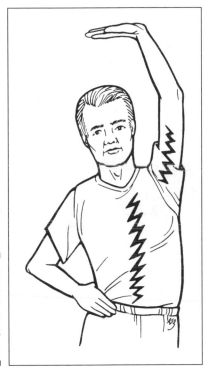

Figure 15-14:
Side stretch
to stretch
the muscles
of your back
and sides.

1. **Stand up straight, with your feet shoulder-width apart and pointing directly forwards. Place the palms of your hands on your lower back.**

2. **Gently breathe in and out until you feel relaxed.**

3. **Bend your upper body backwards, supporting your back with your hands and keeping your knees straight.**

   Try exhaling as you lean back.

4. **Hold the arch for a count of five.**

5. **Gradually return to your starting position.**

Repeat three to five times.

Exercise 16: Head roll

This exercise gently stretches the neck muscles. You get more of a stretch if you hold your shoulders still and don't bring them up to your ears.

1. **Sit on a chair or stand at ease as you hold your head high and look straight ahead.**

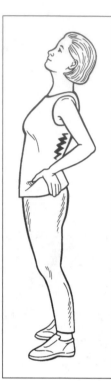

Figure 15-15:
Back arch
to stretch
your
shoulder,
back, and
hip muscles.

2. **Tilt your head to the left as though you were trying to put your ear on your shoulder, as shown in Figure 15-16a.**

   Stop when you have stretched your neck as far as you can. Don't bring your shoulder up to try to meet your ear.

3. **Roll your head forwards and down, as though trying to put your chin on your chest, as shown in Figure 15-16b.**

4. **Continue the roll to the right, as though trying to place your right ear on your right shoulder (Figure 15-16c).**

5. **Come full circle by tilting your head back, as shown in Figure 15-16d.**

   Don't do this if it hurts.

6. **Return to the starting position.**

7. **Repeat these steps in the opposite direction, circling your head to the left.**

Repeat up to five times.

Exercise 17: Head pull

This exercise gently stretches the neck muscles.

1. **Sit in a chair with your back straight and your hands clasped behind your head.**

2. **Gently pull your head forwards and down to stretch the back of your neck, as shown in Figure 15-17.**

3. **Hold, feeling the stretch.**

4. **Return to the starting position.**

Repeat up to five times.

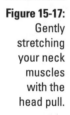

Figure 15-17:
Gently
stretching
your neck
muscles
with the
head pull.

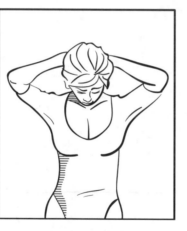

Exercise 18: Neck tilt

Follow these steps to stretch the neck muscles.

1. **Sit or stand comfortably, facing straight ahead.**

2. **Tilt your head to the left, as though trying to put your ear on your shoulder. (Figure 15-18a)**

   Don't try to bring your shoulder up to your ear.

3. **When you feel resistance, hold the position for a few seconds.**

4. **Return to the starting position.**

5. **Repeat in the opposite direction, tilting towards the right. (Figure 15-18b)**

Repeat up to five times.

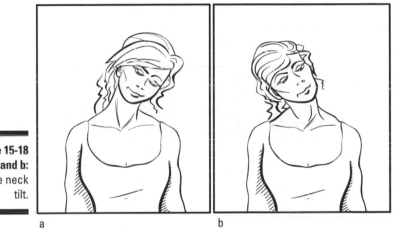

Figure 15-18 a and b: The neck tilt.

a   b

Exercise 19: Shoulder shrug

This exercise stretches both your neck and shoulder muscles.

1. **You can do this lying in bed, or sitting, or standing with your arms at your sides.**

2. **Slowly and steadily raise your shoulders in a shrug (Figure 15-19a).**

3. **Hold for a moment feeling the effect on your neck muscles.**

4. **Keeping your head still, gently press your shoulders down as far as you can (Figure 15-19b).**

5. **Hold, feeling the stretch in your neck.**

Repeat up to five times.

Exercise 20: Shoulder roll

This exercise gently stretches your neck and shoulder muscles and is great as a quick fix for easing tension.

1. **Sit or stand with your shoulders relaxed.**

2. **Raise your shoulders.**

Figure 15-19 a and b: Shrugging your shoulders to ease neck and shoulder stiffness.

a   b

3. **Bring your shoulders forward, as shown in Figure 15-20a.**

4. **Push your shoulders down.**

5. **Pull your shoulders back (Figure 15-20b).**

6. **Return to the starting position.**

7. **Circle your shoulders in the opposite direction, repeating the steps.**

Repeat up to five times.

Cooling down after your exercise programme can help you get ready for the rest of your day. Cool-down exercises can be as simple as taking a short walk for five or ten minutes to keep your muscles loosened up.

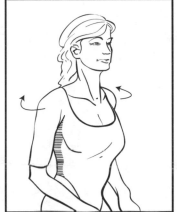

Figure 15-20 a and b: Rolling your shoulders forwards and backwards.

a   b

Chapter 16

Products to Improve Your Back and Neck Health

*T*his chapter covers various postural products – devices that may be helpful for your back or neck pain. All postural products have one important function: To support your spine and extremities in a natural, neutral position. This healthy position lowers the harmful joint stresses that come with poor posture and promote pain relief, recovery from injury, and tolerance to future episodes of spinal pain.

When you stand, you assume a posture that keeps your spine in more of a comfortable, neutral position (refer to Chapter 14). This neutral position is why most people stand up and walk around to find relief from sitting, sleeping, or reclining in poor postures.

When you're not standing, the furniture you use largely dictates your posture. You probably spend the majority of your time off your feet, and so good furniture is important. The posture of your back and neck during rest and activity is your choice – a choice that gives you power over your spinal health.

Postural products come in two basic varieties:

- **Products that support from the ground up:** These products include well-designed office chairs, adjustable beds, and chairs for use at home. These pieces of furniture are adjustable and provide the greatest benefit of all the postural products available. However, generally these products are more expensive than other postural products.

- **Products that enhance support with poorly designed furniture:** These products are mainly portable supports for your lower back and neck. They tend to be affordable and transportable, and may be your only options when you're away from home or work.

In this chapter we group these products by *lifestyle zones* – that is, areas in which each product type comes into play. Thousands of products exist for back and neck pain, and we can't list every product, manufacturer, or retailer. You can buy these products from specialist shops such as Anatomia and The Back Shop (details in Appendix B). Prices are correct at the time of going to press, but are liable to change, so check with the shop before purchasing.

You may wonder how we selected the products we mention in this chapter. Well, we didn't: We asked the people at The Back Shop – a store specialising in products designed for people with back and neck pain – to tell us their most popular items.

Relaxing at Home

Home is where you expect to find relief from the day's stresses. Your home environment, however, can actually increase the stress on your back or neck.

Beware of sofas and chairs that you sink into. This position rounds out your back and brings your chin into your chest. You trade a couple of minutes of early bliss for pain and tightness that cause you to shift and eventually get up. A good guideline to follow is this: You should feel as good, if not better, when you get off your furniture than when you got on it.

Take the opportunity to make your home a place where you have control over the health of your back and neck.

Everyday chairs for the home

These are chairs specifically designed to give maximum support.

- ✔ **Stokke Variable:** This chair stimulates your circulation and helps prevent stiffness (£229).

- ✔ **Stokke Actulum/Pendulum:** This chair promotes natural movement and helps to stimulate your circulation (£325–£367).

- ✔ **Stokke Gravity II:** This all-purpose chair provides maximum relaxation and supports your whole body (£1,142).

- ✔ **The La-Z-Boy Rialto Wall Recliner:** A comfortable, manually operated recliner with a 3-position footrest and multi-position back rest (£506).

Massage chairs

Massage is extremely beneficial for the relief of muscle spasm and can improve circulation in your muscles and joints. Consider trying one of the following massage chairs:

- ✔ **Techno Massage Chair:** This is designed to combine comfort with massage (£1,995).

- ✔ **Optima Massage Chair:** Massaging rollers travel up and down the back of this chair. You can choose from a selection of different levels of massage (£2,995).

- ✔ **Putnams Massage Cushion:** This cushion offers vibrations to refresh your tired back and stiff neck (£15.95).

Sleeping Soundly

Sleep is essential for good health and mental alertness. Back and neck pain are the most common night-time pains, and many people with back or neck pain wake up feeling unrefreshed.

When you sleep, you have no conscious control over your posture and may irritate your back and neck if your mattress gives poor support. A good mattress supports you properly, no matter how many times you move during the night. In this section we describe some products that can support you properly as you sleep.

Mattresses

Many people with back and neck pain find all ordinary mattresses uncomfortable. These specially designed mattresses may help.

- **Back Shop Bed:** This pocket-sprung mattress, with a choice of bases, keeps the body and spine supported, and gives a balance of comfort and support (price on application).

- **Mattress Toper-Obusforme:** This mattress has a temperature-sensitive foam that moulds itself to your body's contours and relieves pressure points (£65–£109).

- **Impression foam mattress:** This mattress adapts to your body. This mattress may be useful for you if you don't have a regular sleep pattern or if you require a high degree of pressure relief (£475–£825).

Pillows

The following pillows are specially designed for people with back and neck pain.

- **Putnams Pillow:** This pillow supports your head and neck and aligns your spine correctly, helping restful sleep. The pillows are available in standard foam and *memory impression foam*, which is temperature-sensitive and moulds itself to your neck, giving pressure relief (£29–£65).

- **Royal Rest Pillow:** This pillow has high and low sides with built-in support cores, giving maximum air circulation (£52).

- **Harley Pillow:** This pillow has a contoured design that supports your head and cervical spine with minimal pressure by gently moulding around you (£62).

- **Obusforme Pillow:** This pillow is made from temperature-reactive memory foam, which gives a gravity-defying feeling: Memory foam responds to the heat and weight of the person sleeping on it (£52).

Opting for Office Comfort

If you sit at a desk for many hours a day, you may experience discomfort and even job dissatisfaction. In this section we suggest some office furniture that can help your back and neck.

Office chairs and stools

Ergonomic office seating has been the focus of much interest in recent years and a variety of products are now available.

More expensive chairs

As you can see, the upper end of the market does not come cheap.

- ✔ **Hag Signet:** This comfortable chair supports you in any position, whether you're leaning backwards or sitting forwards (£2,140).

- ✔ **Hag Capisco:** This chair has a unique seat design that opens up the angle of your hips to comfortably and correctly align your spine (£556).

- ✔ **Hag Credo:** This chair tilts forwards and backwards as you do and remains balanced as you sit upright. An optional headrest is available. (£623.)

- ✔ **Hag HO5:** This ergonomic chair has an adjustable seat depth, height, and forward tilt (£536).

- ✔ **Plus Range:** The workstation chairs in this range are fully adjustable, incorporating a mid-pivotal back support, a floating seat, and inflatable lumbar support (£775–£1,020).

- ✔ **Aeron:** This cross-performance chair is supportive for both computer-related, task-intensive work, and for more relaxed writing and reading (£884).

- ✔ **The RH Logic 4 Elegance:** This smart office chair offers support and healthy postures throughout all your sitting positions and movements (£937).

- ✔ **The Grahl Synchron 7 Duo-Back:** This chair offers comfort, support, and is easily adjustable to fit a wide range of body shapes and sizes (£977).

Medium-priced chairs

Even the medium-priced chairs are hardly inexpensive but worth the investment if you spend a lot of time at your desk.

- ✔ **Vicki Lowback and Highback:** This chair is designed as a stackable conference or reception chair, and features a flexible back and seat to promote dynamic seating (£325–£340).

- ✔ **Bodybilt Petite:** Offers low back support and comfort with posture control at your command (£595).

- ✔ **HO4 CREDO 4470:** Offers support with a tilt function and optional armrests (£245).

Stools

- ✔ **Salli:** This stool provides a balanced posture with your thighs slanting downwards at about 45 degrees. Your pelvis supports your back, leaving your feet and legs less restricted. The height is adjustable (£320).

- ✔ **Dynamic:** The ergonomic seat offers maximum freedom of movement without putting pressure on your back (£599).

Kneeler chairs

- ✔ **Hag Balans Vital:** This chair is the original kneeling chair and offers an alternative seating posture. Most suitable for short periods of sitting, the chair helps your spine adopt an 'S' curve when you're leaning forwards and working at a desk (£320).

- ✔ **Putnams-Kneeler:** You can fold away this height-adjustable kneeling chair when not in use (£130).

- ✔ **Stokke Multi:** This chair promotes the natural curve of your back, leading to a comfortable sitting position. Both the height and the angle of the seat are easily adjustable. The chair folds flat when not in use (£213).

- ✔ **Stokke Wing:** This chair is forward-tilting, with a rocking action, adjustable knee-pads, and height-adjustable gas lift (£413).

- ✔ **Stokke Move:** This height-adjustable chair provides a full 360 degrees of free and easy movement (£215).

- ✔ **Putnams Coccyx Relief Chair:** This chair has the usual kneeler features but also has a coccyx relief recess to take pressure off the base of your spine (£115).

Laptop package

In this computer chair from The Back Shop (£239), you place your keyboard and mouse on a tray attached to an armrest, therefore creating an integrated computer workstation that allows you to sit back, relieving strain on your arms.

Changeable-height workstations

A changeable-height work surface is an optimum tool in your fight against back, shoulder, and neck pain. The Back Shop offers ergonomic space-planning and design tailored to your needs for your office or home. Each design is individually planned to meet your needs and problems.

Ergonomic footrests

An ergonomic footrest, which can lower the occurrence of back problems, is an often-overlooked component to a proper workstation. Most footrest products tilt to keep the feet at a 90-degree angle, thereby enhancing blood circulation. More important, placing your feet on the footrest ensures that you don't slide forwards. An ergonomic footrest lets you sit without having to cross your legs to lock yourself in place, which causes 'rounding' of the lower back and decreases the benefit of your chair.

The Hag Quickstep is an adjustable footrest to help you work more comfortably. You can use this dynamic tool to give your legs a gentle work out and stretch your muscles during your working day (£77).

Travelling in Comfort

Your back or neck pain may cause you to worry about travelling, because of being far away from home and the security of your medical practitioners. With a bit of planning and the right equipment, however, you can begin to enjoy the thought of travelling. Consider some of the following products to make your trips more enjoyable:

- **Putnams wedges and supports:** A wedge can transform a straight horizontal seat into a comfortable, forward-tilting chair. The wedge helps you adopt good posture and maintain the natural curves of your spine by gently rocking your pelvis forwards on your hips (£27–£35).

- **Posture Curve Comfy:** This cushion gently supports your spine and adjacent ligaments and muscles. The cushion is effective both in the home and office and when travelling (£35).

- **Backfriend:** This light, portable back support encourages relaxation of your back muscles by supporting the natural curve of your lumbar vertebrae (£57–£69).

- **Cumfy Coccyx Cushion:** This cushion reduces the pressure from sitting down below your coccyx region (£31.50).

- **Obusforme Travel:** This miniature cervical-support pillow provides supportive comfort and promotes restful sleep. You can also use this cushion as a child's pillow (£31.50).

Staying Fit and Healthy

Exercise is the cornerstone of your body's health – but being safe and sensible is the cornerstone of a safe exercise programme. Plan your exercise programme carefully before you start to ensure that you don't suffer setbacks.

Always check with your doctor before initiating any home therapy or exercise programme, including the use of an exercise ball.

✔ **Fitbox Gymball:** Use this giant, inflatable exercise ball to increase your fitness and mobility by using it as part of your exercise programme in the gym. It is also large enough to be used as a seat to encourage good posture.

✔ **Trimilin Rebouder:** This small, portable trampoline can improve your fitness, stamina, and flexibility. You can take safe and effective vigorous exercise without putting stress and impact on your ligaments and joints.

Part V
Resuming Normal Activity and Preventing Future Injury

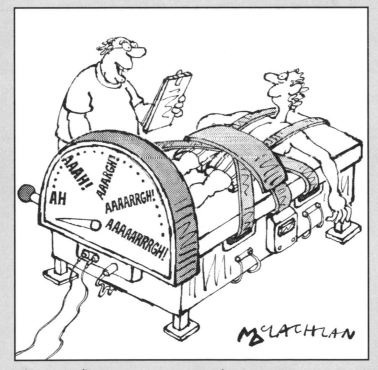

"This is a very simple traction
machine for your back, Mr Wisblister,
— it has only 5 settings."

In this part . . .

*B*ack and neck pain permeates every area of your life, including that intimate, behind-closed-doors part. Sooner or later, though, you will be able to return to *all* your normal activities. Doing so, however, can be harder than you think if you fear re-injury or feel as if you must go to great lengths to protect your back and neck. That's where this part comes in. We tell you how to keep your back and neck healthy and work to diminish your fears as you return to work – and play.

Chapter 17

Getting 'Back' to Work

● ●

In This Chapter

▶ Returning to a risky occupation

▶ Removing roadblocks to your return to work

▶ Planning your return to work

▶ Staying at work after you return

● ●

*R*eturning to work after back or neck pain has kept you from your job can be scary. You may doubt your ability to do your job, especially if your work is physical, and you may wonder whether you're up to spending eight hours at work – not to mention travelling to your workplace – without resting your back or neck.

On the other hand, returning to work can be exciting. Work gives you a sense of purpose and makes your life more normal and routine. Shedding the discomfort and unpredictability of pain may be a relief in itself. Research shows that people who return to work sooner have lower chances of developing chronic pain.

This chapter talks about the pros and the cons of heading back to your job and helps you develop a successful return-to-work plan.

Pondering the Purpose of Work

The average person spends at least a third of his or her day at work. In terms of time commitment, work is likely to be a major part of your life. Work gives you a sense of self-esteem and identity – and of course money. Arguably, the type of work you do identifies you in society more than any other factor.

A back or neck injury that stops you working isn't only a physical blow to your body but also a mental and emotional shock. The longer your back or neck pain keeps you away from work, the more your pain may affect you emotionally and within your social circles.

You're not alone!

Disability due to spinal pain is approaching epidemic proportions worldwide. In the United States, an estimated 5.2 million American adults are disabled by lower-back pain. Of these, approximately half are disabled temporarily and the other half disabled permanently. In the UK in one widely quoted survey, 8 per cent of adults said they had bed rest for back pain at some time in the previous 12 months.

Lower-back pain is the most common cause of disability in the working population under the age of 45 years and the third most common cause of disability in the working population between the ages of 45 and 65 years. Studies show that if you have a lower-back pain disability, you may be out of work longer compared with workers disabled from other injuries.

Studies indicate that if you have been off work because of back pain for about six months, your chances of going back to work are about 75 per cent. After 12 months, those chances decline to 50 per cent. If you have been disabled from work due to back pain for more than two years, your chances of ever returning to work approach zero. Keep in mind, however, that these statistics are based on large groups of injured workers and may not predict what can happen to you as an individual. But knowing these statistics can help ensure that you don't become a 'statistic'.

Neck pain is almost as common as lower-back pain but the consequences are far less devastating: Lower-back pain accounts for approximately ten times the disability, health care use, and state benefit costs of neck pain.

Even when you've been disabled for quite some time because of injury, the tips and suggestions in this chapter can help you get back to some type of work.

Identifying Risky Occupations

In this section, we don't cover specific jobs but rather look at the types of activity that you may perform as part of your job. If you're working on improving your back or neck problem, this section can help you avoid future disability. If you're out of work because of a back or neck injury, try using this information to help you design a successful return-to-work programme.

Jobs that require lifting and bending

When your job requires heavy lifting, pulling, or carrying, the repetitive movements and strain can lead to lumbar disc disease (which we describe in Chapter 3). Many studies show a significant association between lifting, pushing, and pulling and lower-back pain and sciatica.

The posture that you adopt when lifting is particularly important. As we discuss in Chapter 14, lifting and twisting at the same time is one of the worst positions. This type of movement can tear the structures surrounding the discs in your spine. If you lift and twist improperly at work, you have a two- to threefold increase in the risk of lumbar disc herniation.

If your job involves heavy labour, a number of factors increase your chances of having a back or neck injury: Lifting heavy weights, lifting frequently, and lifting with a poor technique. Your overall physical fitness also comes into play. For instance, if you exceed your overall physical capacity for lifting on a regular basis, your risk of lower-back injury increases as much as four times. We discuss a rough guide to lifting in Chapter 14.

Although your maximum lifting load is highly variable depending upon your physical condition, generally the maximum lifting load is 15–20 kilograms (30–35 pounds) for women and 25–30 kilograms (50–60 pounds) for men. If you regularly lift objects that are much heavier than these guidelines, watch out. Consider asking for help or using some other technique, such as a trolley, to avoid lifting.

If you have a job that requires heavy lifting, check out Chapter 14 for information on good posture. Using proper posture and lifting techniques and staying in good physical condition can help prevent spinal injury. (A good back brace may also help; see Chapter 8). If you can't do heavy lifting because of a back or neck injury, you need to decide whether you're going to be able to return to that type of work. Check out 'Preparing to Return to Work' later in this chapter for more information.

All shook up: Exposure to vibration

Prolonged exposure to vibration, especially caused by motor vehicles, increases your risk of lower-back and neck pain, sciatica, and disc herniation. The frequency of vibration that is stressful to your back and neck is similar to the vibration you experience when travelling in a car. According to studies, if you're exposed to vibration during work, your risk for developing one of these conditions is two to three times that of the general population.

You're at greater risk for a back or neck injury when you travel more than 20 miles a day to work or drive a lorry as part of your working day. If you spend more than half your job driving a motor vehicle, you're three times more likely than the average worker to suffer a herniated disc.

Commuting

Commuting by car, bus, train, or underground means you're in a sitting position as your spine is subjected to vibration. Try following these tips to protect your back and neck as you travel:

✔ **Watch your position:** Use the information on healthy posture in Chapter 14 to make sure that your sitting position is upright and your pelvis tucked back. Move your seat up so that you can easily reach the car pedals without stretching your legs. Reclining the backrest about 5–15 degrees can also be helpful.

✔ **Do some easy commuter stretches:** When you're stationary in the car (at traffic lights for example), occasionally push your arms straight on the steering wheel to help decompress your lower back and pelvis. You can also periodically arch your lower back forwards and away from the back of the seat while doing a slight stretch.

✔ **Check your seat:** Check your seat to see whether you need better back support; if necessary, use a lumbar roll (a foam roll for

lumbar support), and if possible reposition yourself and the seat. You can also take the weight off your spine by using an armrest. Many people with neck pain find a neck support helpful.

✔ **Avoid keeping your head turned to one side:** As you travel, avoid keeping your head turned to one side for longer than five minutes. This position can cause muscle tension in your neck and lower back. If you do notice tension from turning your head, look in the opposite direction for a few seconds to help balance yourself out.

✔ **Stay relaxed:** Travelling in stop-and-go traffic can make you tense. To combat stress, try playing relaxing music or listening to a book on tape, or take a few deep breaths, exhaling slowly each time (we discuss breathing exercises in Chapter 13).

✔ **Take breaks on a long drive:** If you're driving for a long time, take breaks every 30–45 minutes and get out of the car.

A sitting position places additional stress on your spine (as we explain in Chapter 14). As your spine is exposed to vibration in the sitting position when driving, your spine is exposed to greater stress. Vibration also fatigues the muscles that support your spine.

When your job exposes you to excessive vibration, you can take steps to reduce vibration to your spine by driving a car with better suspension, avoiding driving over rough terrain, using proper posture (as we discuss in Chapter 14), and using a seat cushion and/or back brace that provides proper support. If you're out of work from a job that exposes you to vibration, you need to take special steps to return safely to that type of work. For more about returning to work, see 'Identifying What's Stopping You from Returning to Work' later in this chapter.

Sitting down on the job

You're at an increased risk of back or neck injury when your job requires you to sit down a great deal. Sedentary occupations in general aren't good for your spine because sitting puts pressure on the discs between your vertebrae.

If you feel you're chained to your desk, use a few techniques to prevent injury: Adopt correct posture, take frequent breaks, follow a back-stretching programme (which we describe in Chapter 15), and at least try to limit your overall sitting time.

Check out Chapter 14 for more details on what you can do to prevent injury from sitting for long periods.

Identifying What's Stopping You from Returning to Work

Even though you may be motivated to return to work after a lower-back or neck injury, other factors may cause difficulty:

- ✔ **Legal intervention:** Legal aspects involved in your work injury case can act as an obstacle to returning to work. Legal action often creates an adversarial relationship between you and your employer. You may consciously or unconsciously believe that returning to work is going to damage your legal case, which ultimately affects your ability to return successfully to work.

- ✔ **Job dissatisfaction:** Research indicates that how much you like (or don't like) your job may be one of the most important risk factors for getting a back or neck injury that results in disability. This finding makes sense: The more enjoyable and satisfying your job, the more motivated you are to return to work, regardless of your pain.

- ✔ **Unemployment benefits:** The type and amount of sick pay you receive may affect your return to work. If your sick pay closely approximates your normal take-home pay, you're likely to be out of work longer after a back or neck injury. If you're not receiving enough money to support yourself while out of work because of a spinal injury, you're more likely to return to any type of work in order to support your family.

- ✔ **Psychological factors:** Occupational stress, job dissatisfaction, anxiety, and depression are all risk factors for spinal injury and pain. These same psychological factors can delay or prevent your return to work after injury.

✔ **Inappropriate medical care:** Receiving inappropriate treatment for your spinal problem can delay your return to work. Examples of inappropriate care include too much bed rest, inactivity, or over medication.

✔ **Chronic health problems:** Other concurrent health problems, in addition to your spinal injury, can mean that you're less likely to be able to return to work. Your spinal injury may be the final straw in terms of your physical ability to do your job.

✔ **Poor labour market:** A particularly bad labour market in your area can delay your return to work because of a decrease in the number of opportunities, especially if you aren't going to return to your previous job or career.

✔ **Limited education/job skills:** If your education is limited and your jobs have always been in heavy physical labour, you may have difficulty returning to work after a significant spinal injury.

Preparing to Return to Work

A *return-to-work programme* may include anything you and your practitioner can do to increase the chances of you returning to work and staying there. You can do some of these things before returning to work and others in the early phases of your return.

Physically reconditioning

Physically reconditioning your body so that you can complete your job is a crucial part of preparing to return to work. When you've been out of work because of a spinal injury, your body may have become physically deconditioned. *Deconditioning* may result in a loss of muscle strength and endurance, decreased aerobic capacity and mobility, and inability to co-ordinate your movements properly. Physical reconditioning prepares your body to do your work activities. If you return to work before your body is physically ready, you increase your chances of having another spinal injury and more disability. The better shape you're in, the more likely you can return to work successfully.

The aerobic efficiency of your body is part of your ability to do your job over an eight-hour day and a 40-hour week. If you've been out of work because of a spinal injury, your aerobic conditioning has probably diminished. Thus, part of your physical reconditioning needs to include aerobic exercise (Chapter 15).

Understanding your limits

Being a knowledgeable worker is your most important safeguard against re-injury. Understand your capabilities, how to work safely, and when you need to refrain from an activity at work that may cause re-injury. Being knowledgeable in the following areas is extremely important for a successful return to work:

- ✔ **Body mechanics:** *Body mechanics* involve how you position and move your body, especially in relation to your spine (we discuss these issues in Chapter 14). Using proper, safe body mechanics helps decrease the stress on your spine and prevent re-injury.

- ✔ **Pacing:** To pace yourself, take regular breaks throughout your working day in order to prevent a build-up of stress on your spine. For example, when your job requires extended sitting, take regular breaks to stand up, walk around, and do some stretching exercises. When your job requires bending and lifting, you need to take regular breaks from that activity.

- ✔ **Setting limits:** When you return to work, set appropriate limits based on your physical capabilities to protect your spine. You can limit the amount of bending, lifting, and twisting you do, and also the amount of repetitive spinal movements done at any one time.

Sometimes setting limits can be difficult when your supervisor is requesting you to complete a certain task 'as quickly as possible'. At these times you must be assertive and protect your spine and prevent re-injury. Doing a task quickly to save a few minutes isn't worth risking another episode of disability.

Preparing for flare ups

After you return to work, you can usually expect flare ups in your spinal pain due to the increased physical demands on your body. Therefore, anticipate these flare ups so that you aren't surprised or too concerned if they do occur. Use some of the suggestions in Chapters 8 and 15 to help you successfully get through the flare up phase. Returning to part-time work with restrictions can also help prevent a serious flare up or setback.

Discuss with your GP any flare up that seems to go beyond something temporary. A common pattern we see in patients who return to work is three steps forwards but one step back: Your work abilities and spinal pain may improve, followed by a slight regression. Don't be concerned if you notice this common pattern.

Returning to the Office

When you work in an office, sitting for long periods and bending over certain office equipment exposes your spine to stress. If you work in this type of environment, pay attention to the good posture rules we discuss in Chapter 14. In addition, you can try the following ideas:

- **Avoid keeping your head down:** When sitting at your desk or computer terminal, or when standing over the copy machine, avoid the head-down position for an extended period of time. Pointing your head down places your neck and back in an unhealthy position.

- **Reposition yourself frequently:** Reposition yourself to a healthy position frequently. We discuss healthy sitting positions in Chapter 14 and suggest pushing your pelvis back in your chair, using a chair that supports your spine, and not crossing your legs excessively.

- **Stretching at your desk:** In addition to the stretching exercises discussed in Chapter 15, take a short break every once in a while and perform the following stretching exercises:

  - **Pelvic rocking** involves taking a deep breath through your nose and stretching your body in the directions indicated by the arrows in Figure 17-1. Position your body upwards and tuck your chin towards your chest. Exhale through your mouth while relaxing after the stretch. Do this exercise every 30–60 minutes when sitting.

  - **Forward stretching** is useful if muscle tension from sitting too long makes your back or neck uncomfortable. To do this exercise, sit up in a tall, relaxed, upright manner with your hands on your thighs to take the weight off your spine. Breathe in through your nose as you adopt this position, stretching yourself tall and in the directions of the arrows shown in the first picture of Figure 17-2. As you exhale through your mouth, allow your head gradually to release forwards. As your head releases forwards, think of the bones of your spine as the links of a chain. Allow each link to release sequentially, one at a time, from top to bottom, as in the second picture in Figure 17-2. Stop lowering your body when you feel ready to inhale or when you achieve an adequate stretching sensation in your back, as in the third picture in Figure 17-2. At this point, release your body a little bit further as you inhale and then exhale again.

    Continue this breathing pattern, releasing your body a little bit further each time you exhale. You should feel a release of tension in your neck, middle back, and lower back. Ultimately, you can reach the position, as shown in the fourth picture in Figure 17-2. Hold this position for a few moments before slowly returning to the upright position.

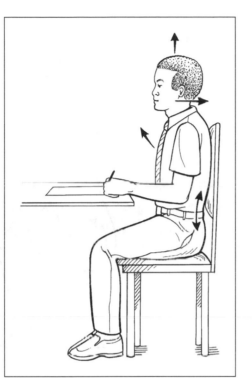

Figure 17-1:
Stretching
your upper
body in the
direction
of the
arrows to
experience
pelvic
rocking.

This exercise may cause temporary changes in your blood pressure, making you feel dizzy. We suggest you don't stand up immediately after doing this exercise.

- **Spine release rotation** is another good exercise to do as you sit at your desk. After doing the forward stretch that we describe in Figure 17-2, bring one arm to the outside of the opposite knee and turn so that you can reach your other arm over the back of your chair. (See the first picture in Figure 17-3.) Gently turn your head, shoulders, and spine as far as you comfortably can in this same direction. Do this movement while keeping your knees straight ahead. You should feel a comfortable and gentle stretch of your back. Don't worry if you notice little clicking sounds coming from your spine – these are normal. Each time you exhale, let your arms twist your back a little further, as feels comfortable. After you inhale and exhale between one and three times, unwind slowly to the front position. Repeat the process in the opposite direction, as in the second picture in Figure 17-3.

This is a gentle stretch and is not to be done to the point of pain or discomfort.

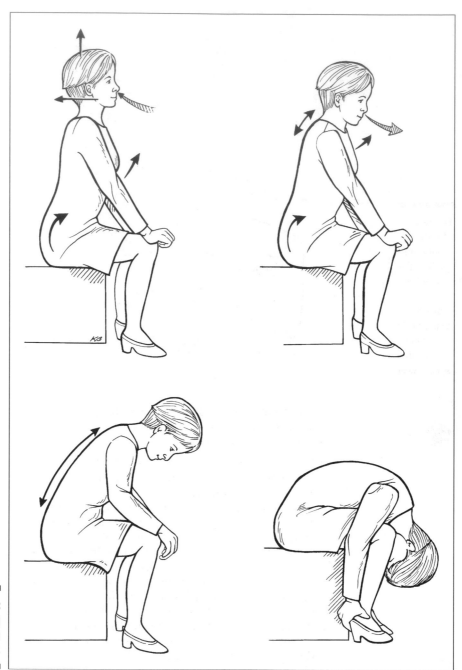

Figure 17-2:
Stretching
while sitting
in a chair.

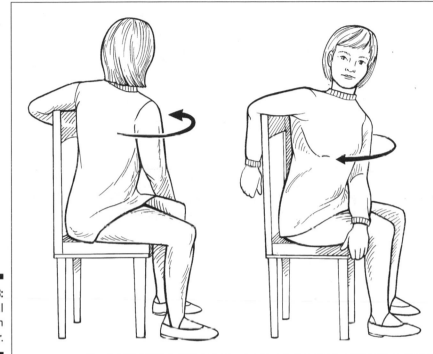

Figure 17-3:
Rotational
stretching in
your chair.

Chapter 18

Returning Safely to Your Favourite Sports

In This Chapter

▶ Reaping the benefits of sporting activities

▶ Enjoying sport even when you have back or neck pain

▶ Being sensible about your sporting activities

*E*xercise is good for your spine, and playing sport is one of the best ways to get exercise:

✔ Sport provides you with recreation and enjoyment.

✔ Sport is good for your overall general physical health.

✔ Sport is good for your mental condition, improving your concentration and sleep, and decreasing negative emotions such as depression, anxiety, and anger.

✔ Sport usually has a social component, which can provide a distraction from your spinal pain.

✔ Sport increases your chances of taking regular exercise: Meeting a friend for a sporting activity makes you accountable for being there. Although solitary exercise programmes are good for your body and general health, many people find they lack the excitement and sociability of sport.

Unfortunately, sporting activities are among the first things to suffer after you develop back or neck pain problem. You may be afraid of re-injury or feel that your spine can't take the pressure of sport. Stopping your sporting activities, and exercise in general, can lead to *deconditioning syndrome*, which we discuss in Chapter 3, and the associated depression, sleep disruption, muscle weakness, and more back or neck pain.

In this chapter, we discuss some methods to help you return to sporting activities, even if you have ongoing spinal pain. We also discuss some of the specific sports in relation to your pain.

Getting Involved in Sport Safely

You can do many things when playing sport to increase your safety and decrease the risk of injury to your spine. Some sporting activities carry more risk of injury to your spine than others, but the benefits associated with playing sport far outweigh the risks of injury. In this section, we discuss how to stay safe when taking part in sport.

Warming up and cooling down

Before playing sport, always warm up and then do some warm-up stretches. After the game, make sure that you cool down and then do some cool down stretches.

The warm up

Regardless of whether you have back or neck pain, your body needs to warm up before you engage in any sporting activity. Warming up prepares you for the increased physical stress that your body is about to experience.

When you warm up, your heart rate and circulation increase. This allows your muscles to react quickly without straining.

You can warm up in a variety of ways: Try walking, gentle cycling on a stationary bike, or spend some time on a treadmill. Warming up for five to ten minutes is an excellent precursor to participation in sport.

Set an easy, unhurried pace during your warm-up. At the end of your warm-up session, your heart rate should be slightly elevated and you should be sweating a little.

The warm-up stretch

After you warm up, you're ready to begin stretching. We talk you through some good stretching exercises in Chapter 15. Warming up is crucial to being able to stretch your muscles to their limits without strain. If you try to stretch out before warming up, you risk injuring your muscles from the stretching activity.

The focus of your stretching programme depends on the type of sport you are about to engage in. Concentrate your stretching programme on the parts of your body that are going to be under the most stress as you play. For instance, before playing a racquet sport, focus on stretching the muscles of your arms, legs, shoulders, and lower back.

To ensure that you stretch in a healthy and safe manner, follow these guidelines:

- ✔ **No bouncing:** Don't bounce as you stretch in order to increase your range of motion: Bouncing may injure your muscles. Instead, stretch a particular muscle group to the end of its range and then hold the position. Your muscle should 'pull' as you stretch, but never hurt or tear.

- ✔ **Go slowly:** Do your stretching exercises slowly and gradually, and always exhale as you stretch. Hold each stretch for a minimum of 20 seconds and a maximum of 60 seconds.

The cool down

After you finish your activity, remember to cool down. The cool down is probably the most neglected area of safe sport. Cooling down after sport returns your body gradually to its usual resting state, and allows your heart rate, circulatory system, muscle tension, and respiration to return to normal slowly and naturally. Examples of good cool down activities include light walking, slow biking, and gentle swimming.

The cool down stretch

Your muscles contract when you engage in strenuous activity. Lactic acid can build up in your muscles and cause muscle pain if not given a chance to dissipate. When you do your cool down stretch, contracted muscles return to normal, and lactic acid is carried away. The cool down stretch also helps prevent muscle pain later on. You can gently stretch your neck, lower back, and legs (refer to Chapter 15).

Considering competition in your sport

The competitive aspect of sport may be an important issue in keeping your spine safe from injury. If you're a highly competitive person, you may be more likely to sustain a spinal injury or cause a flare up in your pain during a sporting activity.

The movements that often result in spinal injuries and pain flare ups are those in which you go for the heroic 'big play' of the game. For example, a tennis ball may be outside of your normal range of movement, but you decide to go for it rather than conceding the point. Participating in sport safely when you have a spinal problem means letting these kinds of shots go. Think in terms of reserving your energy for other shots throughout the game. You end up doing better overall and decrease the risk to your spine.

Cumulative versus acute effects

The effects of a movement can be cumulative or acute. *Cumulative* means that repeating a particular movement increases its effect. Examples of cumulative effect or injury include the hyperextension of a tennis serve, a wrist or forearm injury due to the motion of bowling, and a lower-back problem exacerbated by the repeated twisting motion of a golf swing.

An *acute effect*, or injury, occurs after a single event – for example, a quick movement outside your normal range of movement without warming up – which causes a muscle strain. An acute injury may be caused by reaching for a tennis shot just outside your normal range, trying a skating move that causes you to fall on your bottom and lower back, or attempting to lift a weight beyond your physical capabilities.

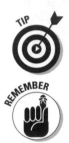

Ask professional coaches or trainers for their advice on getting fit. A lesson with a pro may well be a good investment. Look in Yellow Pages or your local sports centre for details of personal trainers.

Playing when you're physically and/or mentally fatigued is another risk factor with sport. Unfortunately, the weekend athlete follows this pattern: If you work and think hard Monday to Friday, you may be physically and mentally tired on Saturday morning. Pay particular attention to warming up and cooling down when playing weekend games.

Knowing the risks

Understanding the potential pitfalls of a particular sport can be very helpful. Four basic types of movement and posture can exacerbate your spinal pain. You probably use these positions throughout the course of your normal day, but they may become risky if you perform them excessively or repetitively. Look out for the following movements and postures:

- **Flexion:** This movement is bending forwards from a standing position. Flexion puts additional stress on the discs of the lumbar region of your spine.

  Think about how many times during the course of a tennis game you have a choice of bending from the waist (flexion) to pick up the ball or bending your knees properly. The effects of repeated flexion can be cumulative – in other words, the stress of bending over 40 or 50 times to pick up the ball during the course of a game can aggravate your disc problem.

✔ **Extension:** This movement is the opposite of flexion – arching or bending backwards. Excessive extension movements put stress on the facet joints of your lower back because when you arch backwards, the facet joints in your lower back are brought closer together.

As with flexion, the results of repeated extension can be cumulative. For example, your tennis serve involves repeated hyperextension as you throw the ball up and arch your back. You may not notice the effects of a single serve, but 30 or 40 serves can increase your spinal pain.

✔ **Rotation:** Rotating and twisting motions are key movements in a number of sports. Imagine an invisible line passing vertically through the centre of your body, from your head to your buttocks. Now imagine your body, especially between your neck and your hips, is twisting around that imaginary line – this is rotation. Twisting places increased stress on the discs of your lower spine. Although twisting movements are involved in many activities, from ballet to basketball and beyond, you can usually develop techniques to keep this type of movement to a minimum.

✔ **Lifting:** Any lifting places increased stress on your spine, especially if you use a flexion movement, which we describe earlier in this list. Two important components of proper lifting techniques include keeping the object you're lifting as close to your body as possible and bending your knees while using your thigh muscles to bear as much of the weight as possible. Some sports involve more lifting than others, and you can't always follow proper lifting rules when you're playing: Bowling, for instance, requires you to lift a heavy ball and swing it away from your body. Follow proper lifting techniques as best you can and make sure that you warm up and cool down.

Playing Sport with Spinal Pain

In this section, we discuss a number of common sporting activities, starting with sports with the least risk for spinal problems and finishing with sports that have the greatest risk for spinal problems. Table 18-1 shows how we divide up the sports discussed in this section by risk.

Assessing the risk for a particular sport is highly subjective and influenced by a number of factors apart from the sport itself. The intensity with which you participate in the sport also determines how hazardous the sport is to your back and neck: A big difference exists between shooting a few baskets and engaging in a full-court competitive netball game.

Table 18-1		Risk Levels for Spinal Problems Associated with some Common Sports		
Low	*Low to medium*	*Medium*	*Medium to high*	*High*
Cycling	Aerobics	Netball	Golf, bowling	Football
Swimming	Jogging	Racquet sports	Skating	Gymnastics
Dance	Skiing	Weightlifting	Horseback riding	Rugby

Low-risk sports

Cycling, swimming, low-impact aerobics, and dancing pose only a low risk for injury to your spine.

Cycling

Whether you cycle indoors on a stationary bike or outdoors on the open road, you can generally consider cycling to be a low-risk sport for your spinal problem. If you jogged before developing spinal pain but find it difficult to resume running, cycling may be a good substitute.

Cycling provides you with excellent leg exercise, cardiovascular stimulation, and (unless you're on a stationary bike) the experience of being outdoors without the repeated jarring associated with jogging and running. The only way to irritate your spine on a bicycle is by riding on a high seat and using low handlebars so that you hyper-flex your lumbar spine and place stress on the various parts of your spine. Adjust your seat height downwards so that your knee is slightly bent when at full extension on the lower pedal. And remember that mountain biking is rougher on your back than the smooth terrain of road work.

If you experience sciatic pain when cycling, take frequent breaks.

Five to ten minutes on a stationary bike can be an excellent way to warm up before stretching and engaging in other sports.

Swimming

In general, swimming is a very safe exercise and can be excellent therapy for spinal pain. Swimming works almost all your muscles and provides cardio-vascular conditioning. Being in the water protects your spine because the buoyant properties of water provide support and force you to move slowly and smoothly.

Pay attention to the swimming strokes you use: Generally, strokes done on your front, such as breast stroke and front crawl, are more stressful for your back because you're in a position of hyperextension, with your back arched. Butterfly stroke is particularly irritating to your spine because it requires you to flex and extend. Probably the safest and most beneficial swimming strokes are backstroke and side-stroke. Experiment with different styles to see which you find most comfortable.

As with any exercise programme, always warm up and stretch before swimming.

Dancing and aerobics

The physical intensity of dancing and aerobics varies depending on whether you're doing ballet or the twist or practising more sedate styles such as waltzing and ballroom dancing. Equally, high-impact aerobic routines are more stressful than low-impact programmes and may lead to a flare up of your pain.

Slow ballroom dancing is in the very low risk category, but avoid dipping if you have a facet problem (which we describe in Chapter 3), and don't tango if hyperextension causes you more back pain. Higher risk dancing tends to be the more physically demanding stuff, such as swing dancing.

Try to follow these guidelines to make your dancing and aerobics safe and rewarding, even if you have spinal pain:

- ✔ Follow a good general conditioning exercise programme in addition to dancing (refer to Chapter 15 for an exercise programme).
- ✔ Pace yourself when dancing, doing aerobics, or practising your routines.
- ✔ Avoid any movements that obviously aggravate your pain.
- ✔ Remember to warm up and stretch before dancing or doing aerobics.

Low- to medium-risk sports

Participating in the following activities carries some risks to your spine, but with attention and care you can enjoy these sports.

Jogging and running

Under this heading we include everything from speed-walking to sprinting. The bumping and jarring of your feet hitting the road transmits directly to your spine and can aggravate your lower back or neck pain. You can, however, do several things to minimise these forces:

✔ **Warm up and cool down.** Always remember to warm up and stretch before you start running, and then cool down and stretch afterwards.

✔ **Begin gradually.** If you're a novice jogger, start out slowly. Run at a slow speed and go only a short distance until you build up your endurance and get in shape.

✔ **Wear good shoes.** One of the most important ways to decrease the impact of road vibration is to invest in a good pair of shoes. Appropriate running shoes provide excellent support for your feet and absorb some of the jarring shocks to your knees, legs, and lower back. A good guideline is to change your shoes every 150 miles or six months, whichever comes first.

✔ **Run on soft, smooth, flat surfaces.** Running on a grass field or gravel track is much easier on your spine than running on concrete or asphalt. Running on a flat surface causes the least amount of stress to your spine. Running uphill puts your lower spine into a position of flexion as you bend forwards. Running downhill puts extra stress on your spine because you're in a posture of extension, arching backwards.

By using these guidelines, you can safely enjoy some level of jogging while keeping your symptoms of back or neck pain under control and avoiding re-injury.

Skiing

You may be surprised that we mention skiing as a possible sport for people with spinal pain. Skiing, however, is not a bad exercise for your spine, and falling over when skiing rarely causes spinal injuries. In this section, we focus primarily on downhill skiing, although similar issues apply to cross-country skiing.

The common skiing stance – hips and knees flexed, with the body weight forwards – actually protects your lower back. The primary risk of exacerbating your spinal pain due to skiing is falling over or the repeated twisting motion while skiing down the mountain as the top of your body faces one direction and your lower body goes another.

Try following these pointers to make skiing a safe activity, even with spinal pain:

✔ **Warm up and stretch first.** Warming up and stretching is particularly important before skiing. Not only is the outside temperature likely to be cold, but also your body may be subjected to unexpected movements as you negotiate obstacles that seem to come out of nowhere.

✔ **Strengthen your leg muscles.** In your pre-ski strengthening programme, pay attention to developing your *quadricep muscles* (the muscles running from your hips to the front of your knees). These muscles are critical shock absorbers for your entire body when you're skiing and can absorb much of the jarring that normally affects your spine – but only if they're strong enough.

✔ **Avoid twisting.** Avoid twisting your shoulders and hips in opposite directions. Keep your shoulders and hips as parallel as possible to lessen the stress on your lower back.

✔ **Don't ski when you're fatigued.** Most ski accidents occur at the end of the day when skiers are tired and not concentrating on safe techniques. You're more likely to avoid a spinal injury if you stop skiing at the first sign of fatigue.

✔ **Start gradually and lower your sights.** Whether you're just starting to ski or returning to skiing after a spinal pain episode, start gradually and proceed slowly. If you're an advanced skier, start back on the intermediate slopes. Put aside your ego as you build up to your normal level of expertise.

✔ **Watch the ski conditions.** Avoid bumps and obstacles, choose well-groomed ski runs, avoid deep powder snow, and watch out for icy conditions that make for a hard fall. (We suggest you also avoid skiing off 20-foot cliffs while doing flips!)

Medium-risk sports

By taking the proper precautions, you can enjoy netball, racquet sports, and weightlifting

Netball

Experts don't agree about the degree of risk to your spine when you play netball. As with any activity, how you play the game determines the level of risk to your back and neck. If you casually shoot baskets, you're at low risk of hurting your spine. Conversely, if you play a full-court competitive game as part of a league, your risk of injury is greater.

Netball movements associated with spinal injuries include a variety of things such as twisting, extension, flexion, and running. Keep these risk factors under control by paying attention to your approach to the game: As with any other sport, always warm up and stretch before playing and make sure that you play within your range of physical ability, expertise, and safety relative to your pain – you may need to adjust your level of competitiveness.

Racquet sports

Under this heading, we include tennis, racquet ball, squash, and badminton. The primary risk in all these sports comes from twisting your body during the game and while carrying out various shots: serves, overhead smashes, backhands, and lunges.

Follow these guidelines to avoid spinal problems when playing racquet sports:

- ✔ **Adjust your style.** If you have back or neck pain, adjust your serve, overhead shots, and backhand. Consider taking lessons from a professional who can help you adjust your style to avoid hyperextension and excessive twisting.

- ✔ **Stay in shape.** Keep in good overall conditioning and always warm up before playing. Racquet sports tend to be quite social, so you may be tempted to omit your warm-up exercises. But remember: Not warming up increases your risk of exacerbating your spinal pain.

- ✔ **Keep warm.** If you play outdoors in chilly weather, make sure that you dress warmly. If you're cold, you're more prone to pain and discomfort so adequate clothing is essential.

- ✔ **Don't lunge.** The temptation to get that tough shot depends on your level of competitiveness, but lunging for a shot is probably the most frequent cause of spinal injury during racquet sports. Don't do it! Let the shot go and make up points later in the game. You probably perform better overall – and protect your spine.

- ✔ **Try doubles.** If you have severe spinal pain or are returning to a racquet sport after a spinal injury, consider playing doubles. Doubles is easier on your spine because you're less likely to move beyond your normal range of motion.

- ✔ **Wear good shoes.** Wearing proper supportive footwear when playing racquet sports helps decrease the jarring motion on your spine and provides extra support for your feet.

- ✔ **Consider using a back brace.** If you have chronic back or neck pain or you're returning from a back or neck injury, consider wearing a back brace as you play racquet sports. A brace supports and protects your back as you get in shape. We discuss braces in Chapter 8.

- ✔ **Consider your type of racquet.** Many different racquet types are available. Consider purchasing a racquet that absorbs the most shock when contacting the ball and provides the greatest reach. Ask a professional to recommend some racquets.

Weightlifting

Weightlifting puts immense stress on your lumbar spine. Studies show that evidence of spine damage runs as high as 40 per cent among young weightlifters – much higher than in the general population.

The amount of stress placed on your spine depends on the type and intensity of weightlifting you do. Because weightlifting is the cause of so many spinal injuries, see your doctor immediately if you have an increase in pain after weightlifting.

To make your weightlifting safer, follow these tips:

- **Develop your technique.** As with all sports, you can lift weights safely or in a more dangerous manner. Develop your technique and train adequately in order to be safe. Start weightlifting under the guidance of a qualified trainer. And don't try to increase your weight too rapidly or beyond the capabilities of your body.

- **Watch your movements.** The series of movements in typical weightlifting can be stressful on your spine: You flex your back when you pick up a barbell from the ground, stand erect as you bring the weight to your chest, and then hyperextend as you raise the weight over your head. Consult a trainer to ensure safety.

- **Try weightlifting that spares your spine.** When working with a trainer, develop a weightlifting routine that spares your back. Focus on routines that don't place excessive stress on your spine – your trainer can advise you.

- **Wear a weightlifting belt.** A weightlifting belt stabilises your lower spine and protects the muscles of your abdomen. The belt diminishes the strain on that entire area of your body. You can find weightlifting belts at most sports stores.

- **Stay within your means.** Stay within your abilities relative to the amount of weight you're lifting. One way to protect your spine is to lift lighter weights and increase the number of repetitions. Again, working with a qualified trainer can help you develop a safer routine.

Medium- to high-risk sports

Medium- to high-risk sports require more careful attention and using safer techniques because of the increased risk to your spine. Even so, take appropriate precautions and you can still enjoy bowling, golf, and skating.

Bowling

Depending on who you talk to, bowling is rated anywhere from a low- to a high-risk sport. We believe that the threat to your spine from bowling depends on your technique, and so we classify bowling as a medium- to high-risk sport.

Two aspects of bowling can cause problems for your spine: First, the twisting motion you use as you throw the ball – your shoulders and upper torso twist in one direction and your hips and legs twist in the opposite direction. Second, before you throw your strike, you flex your back and hold the heavy ball at arm's length, a position and motion – especially given the weight of the ball – that may irritate your spine, especially the discs and facet joints (which we describe in Chapter 2).

Try following these guidelines to help you bowl without causing more problems for your spine:

- ✓ **Develop a good technique.** One of the best ways to avoid spinal problems when bowling is to develop a good technique. If you have chronic spinal pain and plan to bowl regularly, get an evaluation occasionally from a bowling professional to ensure that your technique is safe for your spine.

- ✓ **Use an appropriately sized ball.** Don't use a ball that is too heavy for you and make sure that the ball fits your fingers well. Ensure that you can manage the weight of the ball while releasing it smoothly and easily from your hand.

- ✓ **Do strengthening exercises.** If you're a regular bowler with a spinal pain problem, doing strengthening and stretching exercises consistently is extremely important to prevent re-injury or acute flare ups. If you rarely bowl, take things easy when you go bowling. The out of condition, occasional bowler with an unsound technique is most at risk of experiencing a spinal problem.

- ✓ **Consider wearing a corset.** Consider wearing a lumbar corset while you bowl, especially after an acute flare up of a chronic back problem. This can support you and remind you to be careful. Of course, don't rely on the corset to the exclusion of stretching, strengthening, and conditioning. See Chapter 8 for more on corsets.

Golf

Spinal problems are the bane of golfers. The twisting motion of the golf swing causes significant stress on the discs and facet joints (which we talk about in Chapter 2), especially if you have a tendency to arch your back extensively through the swing and try to shift your hips 'through the ball' as you hit.

Following these golfing guidelines may help you enjoy your game even if you have spinal pain:

- ✔ **Make sure that you warm up.** Given the highly social component of golf and the fact that it doesn't seem like a strenuous exercise, many golfers don't warm up properly. But, in addition to sand and water hazards, golf includes spinal hazards, which makes warming up and stretching out important before you play.

- ✔ **Develop a safe swing.** Certain swing movements – such as severely arching your back as you hit the ball – can put extra stress on your spine. Consider having a golf professional help you develop a swing that causes the least amount of stress on your spine.

- ✔ **Take care after long absences.** Many golfers don't get in much golfing time during the winter months. Come springtime, you may want to run out to the driving range and hit buckets of balls in order to get back into the game as quickly as possible. However, after a season of inactivity, you may be vulnerable to a spinal problem because your body isn't properly prepared to re-enter the sport. Pay attention to proper conditioning exercises as you ease back into play.

- ✔ **Respect your driver and long irons.** Your back is probably most at risk when you use your driver and long irons and you're likely to utilise a full golf swing with maximum effort, putting more stress on your spine. When hitting with these clubs, pay particular attention to swinging smoothly and easily. Try deciding mentally to hit the ball 10 or 20 metres shorter than usual. You may actually end up hitting the ball farther and more accurately.

- ✔ **Stay warm if you use a golf cart.** Riding in a golf cart essentially lets your body cool down between each golf shot. Instead, try to walk at least a little between shots. And don't forget to dress warmly on cooler days.

- ✔ **Wear soft-spiked shoes.** Many golf courses now require you to wear soft-spiked golf shoes. Wearing this type of shoe may reduce the impact on your spine at the end of your swing. These shoes give you some traction but don't make your stance nearly as solid as regular golf shoes.

Horseback riding

The spinal risk associated with horseback riding involves the vertical impact or bumpy up-and-down motion in the saddle that jars your spine. Also, horseback riding involves primarily the sitting position, which puts a greater load on your spine and discs.

If you're recovering from a spinal injury, consider stopping horseback riding until your pain is minimal or has gone for several months and you've had a chance to recondition your body.

Don't forget the cool down after golf

How many times have you finished 18 holes feeling great, only to wake up the following day with every muscle aching – especially in your back or neck? One likely cause is going straight from the course into a car and sitting in the same position all the way home. You need to cool down after playing any sport, including golf.

After a round of golf, your body is generally supple and warm. If you jump into a car and drive home, your body cools down too rapidly without having a chance to recover from the physical demands of the game.

Try following these tips to cool down after a round of golf:

✔ Go out to the range and hit a few short-iron shots.

✔ Take some time to do some gentle stretching, including your neck, lower back, and legs. (We suggest some good exercises in Chapter 15.)

✔ Take a warm shower.

✔ Don't go immediately from bending over a putt on the 18th green to slumping over an ice-cold drink in the 19th hole.

Use good riding techniques to help ensure that horseback riding doesn't cause a problem for your spine. For instance, with a good riding technique you rarely hit the saddle with any significant impact. As we mention in the section on skiing, your legs need to act as shock absorbers and minimise any impact to your spine. Just as in any sport, stay within your level of expertise and start out gradually if you're a beginner or returning to riding after a spinal problem.

Skating

In this section, we discuss ice-skating, roller-skating, and in-line skating. Skating is generally a medium- to high-risk sport if you have spinal pain, as long as you stay away from stunts and very long strides. Skating is a good form of general exercise and involves smooth, fluid movements, which are just the type of moves you want to make to prevent spinal strain.

Three skating activities can aggravate your spinal condition. Take steps to manage these problems and enjoy skating while keeping your spinal problem under good control:

✔ **The basic skating position** puts your spine in a slightly bent forward position, which can irritate your lower back. Take it easy when skating and stay as upright as possible.

✔ **The spinning motion** associated with ice-skating is perilously close to that twisting motion you need to avoid at all costs.

✔ **Landing after a jump** in ice-skating or in-line skating – including after unplanned falls – isn't healthy for your spine If you have a spinal problem, consider leaving jumps out of your skating routine.

High-risk sports

If you have a back problem, watch out for the sports we describe in this section. These sports are high-risk for starting and exacerbating back pain problems, and you really can't make these sports more spine-friendly. If your involvement in these sports continually causes flare ups of your back or neck pain, you may want to consider pursuing a different activity.

Football and rugby

Football and rugby are high-risk sports, regardless of whether you have spinal pain.

Rugby involves excessive twisting, hyperextension, and weight-bearing. This sport puts stress on your discs, facet joints, muscles, and ligaments (we describe all these in Chapter 2). If you tackle in rugby your back may be flexed more than 45 degrees, and if you're being tackled you may land your spine hyperextended or rotated.

Football is less of a menace than rugby on your back, but it still has the potential to cause problems for your spine, especially if you are a 'weekend athlete' in not particularly good shape or condition.

We suggest that you avoid football and rugby if you have a spinal problem. If you must play, an appropriate strengthening, stretching, and conditioning programme is essential. And always warm up adequately before playing. Ask your doctor for advice on wearing a back brace when playing.

Don't play football or rugby if you have an acute flare up of your pain. If you have a significant flare up after playing, ask your doctor to check your back and neck to see whether you've injured your spine.

Gymnastics

Gymnastics is considered a high-risk sport even if you don't have a spinal pain condition. Some of the spinal stressors involved in gymnastics include the following:

✔ Wear and tear to the facet joints (see Chapter 2 for more on these) from severe hyperextension of the spine.

✔ Strained spinal ligaments from dramatic flexion postures.

✔ Traumatic displacement of a vertebra from fracture due to falling or cumulative effects of certain positions.

The bottom line is that your body isn't designed to extend to the degree required for many gymnastics positions, or to change quickly from a position of full flexion to one of full extension.

Gymnastics is most dangerous for children and teenagers – the group with whom the sport is most popular. A study of young Bulgarian gymnasts showed that 50 per cent of the gymnasts developed spinal problems later in life. If you or your child engages in this sport, pay attention to warming up properly and stretching exercises. Don't push your child to do the movements too quickly.

The risk of spinal injury is great in gymnastics. If you or your child experience prolonged, severe, and unimproved spinal pain after or during gymnastics, seek appropriate medical evaluation and treatment.

Chapter 19

Getting Back in the Saddle: Back and Neck Pain and Sex

*O*ngoing spinal pain can seriously affect your ability to enjoy a sexual relationship. Whether the pain is yours or your partner's, an injured spine can lead to anything from an occasional disruption of sex due to muscle spasm to not having sex for a year or more.

Many of our patients cite sexual problems as one of their primary concerns related to their pain. They often state that none of their other doctors asked them about this aspect of their lives. Pain of any type can disrupt your sexual interactions or, worse, your entire relationship.

Understanding the Vicious Circle of Back and Neck Pain

Frustration, anger, guilt, fear, and depression may all accompany a serious spinal problem. These emotions and the pain itself can almost wipe out any sexual relationship. Spinal pain can both diminish your physical ability to have enjoyable sex and decrease your sex drive.

Spinal pain is invisible, which can cause problems in a couple's physical relationship. If you have spinal pain, you may feel inadequate and have self-critical thoughts such as 'Why would anybody want to sleep with me? I'm unappealing and an invalid.' (See Chapter 13 for more information on negative thoughts.) If you accept these negative thoughts, you may withdraw from sexual interaction.

If you have spinal pain, you might mentally watch, evaluate, and criticise your every sexual move. This can lead to *performance anxiety* – whereby you become so anxious that you no longer enjoy sex and may even avoid it.

If your partner has spinal pain, your thoughts and emotional response to that pain can affect your physical relationship. For instance, you may be afraid of injuring your partner during any sexual interaction and, as a result, you don't initiate sex. If you withdraw from physical interaction, your partner may misinterpret these signals as meaning that you no longer find him or her attractive.

As intimacy dissolves, a vicious circle perpetuates: You and your partner end up moving away from each other physically and emotionally, communicating less, and feeling even more isolated.

Even though spinal pain may limit your ability to perform physically, it doesn't have to limit your overall sexual relationship, which includes mental, emotional, and intimacy aspects. A couple can have a very fulfilling sexual relationship even with a spinal pain problem. To restore your sexual relationship, try to do the following:

- Communicate with each other.
- Focus on sensuality and romance.
- Understand intimacy in your relationship.
- Discover sexual positions that are comfortable for both of you.
- Put in the effort to make the relationship work.

Communicating With Your Partner

The most important aspect of any relationship is good communication. When communication is effective, you usually feel understood and satisfied. When communication breaks down, you may feel embarrassed, unappreciated, misunderstood, defensive, and hostile. All these emotional reactions, positive and negative, are amplified when the issue is sex.

Many people have difficulty talking about sex. When a couple can't communicate openly about their sexual relationship, they create fertile ground for the vicious circle of sex-related problems.

Keep the following hints in mind when communicating with your partner, especially when talking about sex:

- ✔ **Practise listening carefully to each other.** During conversations, most people think about what they are going to say next, rather than focusing fully on hearing the other person. Effective communication involves discovering how to listen attentively to the other person's message. If you really listen, you may gain a full understanding of your partner's thoughts and feelings about an issue. To make sure that you understand your partner, use an *active listening* approach – paraphrase what you think your partner said in order to check for accuracy: After your partner has spoken, say 'So what you're saying is . . . Is that accurate?'

- ✔ **Watch your body language.** When you communicate, make sure that your body language matches your message. Research shows that more than half of what you communicate is conveyed through body language, not words. You may tell your partner that you really enjoy lovemaking, but if you avert your eyes or sigh as you speak, your body language communicates a very different message.

- ✔ **Avoid threatening and judgemental behaviour.** Non-threatening, non-judgemental communication opens the door to meaningful discussion without causing arguments. When the topic is sex, communication that involves no threats or put-downs becomes even more important. The worst way to deal with a sexual problem is to criticise each other, which only fosters defensiveness and hostility.

- ✔ **Respect each other's conversational styles.** Research shows that different communication styles may trigger misunderstandings. Women and men tend to have different communication styles. For instance, women may ask more personal questions and share their feelings and experiences. On the other hand, men may interrupt and dominate a conversation and discuss problems with the sole intent and focus on finding a solution. Other variables, such as your family background, culture, occupation, and education, may also determine your conversational style. Become aware of your partner's style of communication and be respectful of your differences.

- ✔ **Set aside time for communication.** You and your partner must set aside time to communicate about your problems and issues – especially sex. Waiting for the subject to crop up at some point is like having a ticking bomb sitting in your relationship. Try to choose a time for conversation when you and your partner aren't going to be under pressure, rushed, or interrupted.

✔ **Avoid discussing your sex problems in the bedroom.** Mentioning sexual problems during intimacy is a sure-fire way to create problems. Discuss sexual issues outside the bedroom in a non-threatening atmosphere.

✔ **Phrase your comments carefully.** Thinking before speaking is especially important when you're discussing – or considering discussing – sex. Take care to phrase your concerns in a way that doesn't hurt your partner's feelings. Remember, too, that some things are best left unsaid – No one's yet invented something that can retract the spoken word.

✔ **Compliment each other frequently.** Research shows that a very high frequency of negative statements towards each other, relative to the number of positive statements, characterises troubled relationships. When discussing issues – including your sexual relationship – with your partner, stress the positive aspects and phrase your areas of concern in a non-negative way.

✔ **Make your requests specific.** If you want to communicate an issue, be specific and try to do the following:

- **Focus on the behaviour rather than the person:** For instance, don't make global personality statements such as 'You're lazy!' Instead, try using a statement such as: 'It seems to me that you haven't been taking the rubbish out as often as you used to. Is that right?' The second statement addresses the person's behaviour and invites discussion towards finding a solution.

- **Use 'I' rather than 'you' statements:** For instance, notice the difference in the feel of the following statements: 'You didn't buy ice cream at the store because you think that I'm fat!' versus 'When I ask you to buy ice cream at the store and you don't, I feel that you think I'm fat.' The first 'you' statement is accusatory and likely to make the other person defensive. The second 'I' statement communicates the issue but is much softer and invites useful discussion.

✔ **Write a letter.** If you feel shy about sexual communication, try writing your thoughts, feelings, and concerns in the form of a letter to your partner. Letter-writing helps you organise your thoughts and ensure that you present them in a non-threatening manner – and remember to include in the letter plenty of compliments. Writing letters to each other about sexual issues can be an excellent way to overcome the shyness that is often associated with communicating about these issues. You may find that asking your partner to respond with a letter is helpful in getting the communication going.

✔ **Go through this chapter with your partner.** Try reading this chapter together and talking about each section as you go along, or read each section separately and then discuss what you've read with each other. The most important thing is to discuss the information and to practise good communication skills with your partner.

Check to make sure that your partner understands your comments. Ask your partner to paraphrase and summarise what you said or to explain the point you're trying to make. You can then correct any misunderstandings.

Getting in the Mood

A wise person once said 'If there was more courting in marriages, fewer marriages would end up in court.' When spinal pain is an aspect of a couple's sexual relationship, romance and sensuality are more important than ever.

Even if spinal pain is not an issue, the romance and excitement of sex can yield more pleasure than the actual physical activity itself. However, contrary to what films lead us to believe, romance and excitement do not descend from the clouds with a symphony playing in the background. In the real world, communication and planning are usually necessary for romance to occur. Spinal pain doesn't have to interfere with romance and sensuality in your relationship. Try following these tips to set the stage for romance:

- ✔ **Plan a spine-friendly date:** Planning a date or series of dates is a good way to build romance. People with spinal pain sometimes forget that they can still have fun. If your back or neck pain makes you concerned about going on a date, try to plan a sensual romantic interlude that doesn't stress your spine. For example, plan a romantic dinner, an evening swim, or a night away in a hotel. You can add the spontaneity later: Simply planning time together can create sexual excitement as you anticipate the approaching date.

- ✔ **Create a romantic atmosphere:** A romantic setting fosters intimacy that may start many hours or even days before you and your partner become physically intimate. Pay attention to all your senses as you plan, and try to incorporate as many relaxing elements as possible: Try passionate music, soft lighting, delicate incense or potpourri, a delicious dinner, and satin sheets or pyjamas.

- ✔ **Foster emotional intimacy:** Emotional intimacy can begin long before you have sexual contact. Try sending your partner flowers, tucking seductive notes in your partner's bag, or leaving intimate messages on your partner's phone. The possibilities are limited only by your imagination. Emotional intimacy builds the anticipation of your physical encounter, helps you focus on the relationship rather than the spinal pain, and enhances the sensuality of the whole experience.

Getting Physical

Emotional and physical intimacy are intertwined, and they can be fostered by touching, holding hands, hugging, glancing at each other, and using pet names and love talk. After you build up the sensuality, romance, anticipation, and emotional intimacy of your relationship, you're likely to start getting physical. Try the following to create some physical intimacy:

- ✔ Massage your partner, perhaps using massage oils.
- ✔ Soak in a bath together.
- ✔ Kiss each other.
- ✔ Hold hands.
- ✔ Hug your partner.

Physical intimacy may include activities that help you manage your spinal pain more effectively during sex. For instance, many people with spinal pain obtain relief from massage, hot-water bottles, or taking a hot bath. Try incorporating these pain-relieving activities into your intimate activities.

If spinal pain has had a significant impact on your sexual relationship, begin slowly to build sexual activity back into your relationship. Open communication is important and may include planning how you're going to engage in pre-sexual activities and discussing the most comfortable physical positions for the partner with spinal pain.

Sex is exciting, and that excitement can lead to greater physical activity, especially as you approach orgasm. Given this heightened level of physical exertion and focus, you may not notice your spinal pain at the time. Try to keep your level of physical activity under control, especially if you're prone to acute pain flare ups after sex.

Getting Down to It, or Spine-Friendly Sexual Positions

This section outlines some sexual positions that may be comfortable for a person with spinal pain. Experiment with these positions with your partner to find those that work best for both of you. As you try out the positions we describe in this section, remember to take things slowly and communicate openly.

If your spinal pain is severe, try initially to take a more passive role in love-making and pay attention to non-intercourse sexual activity (which we discuss in the following section). Try talking with your partner about your need to be more passive until you work up to being able to tolerate more activity. Discussing this issue openly may make you more comfortable about being passive and help your partner understand that you're not just being selfish.

Getting started

Not all sexual encounters involve genital intercourse. Many people with spinal pain are more comfortable starting out if intercourse is not the goal of physical interaction.

If you have spinal pain, you may find that lying on your back on a firm surface and placing your legs on a pillow is a comfortable position. You may also gain comfort by rolling or folding a small hand towel under your lower back, giving it a slight arch and providing additional support. This position is fairly passive for the person with the pain, but you can still do and gain a lot.

Your search for a firm surface can double as a way to create a romantic atmosphere – try out the lounge floor, the dining-room table, or any other place that takes your fancy.

Outercourse

Pain – or fear of pain – is one of the primary obstacles to sexual pleasure and orgasm, so make sure that you proceed slowly and patiently. You may find genital intercourse too painful at first, so don't make it your initial goal. As you recover from a flare up of pain or adjust to the changed condition of your spine, limit your lovemaking to other forms of sexual interaction done in a relaxed position. The goal is to avoid frustration and any significant increase in pain.

Outercourse – a term we borrowed from *Sex For Dummies* by Dr Ruth K. Westheimer – is a modern term for what we used to call 'heavy petting'. You can be involved in sexual stimulation even from a relaxed position, and either partner can provide manual and/or oral stimulation. In fact, you can provide sexual stimulation in a variety of ways: Try to have fun with your partner exploring the possibilities.

The missionary position

The *missionary position* is basically the male superior position. And no, we aren't referring to any power hierarchy based on gender. Put simply, the man goes on top and the woman underneath. Variations on the missionary position can be useful if you have spinal pain, depending on the type of your pain.

If you're a woman with spinal pain, you may find the missionary position fairly comfortable:

- ✔ Lie on your back with your legs bent, which allows you to maintain some curve in your spine. The degree your spine curves is relative to how close you bring your knees to your chest. If you don't find this traditional missionary position comfortable, place a towel or small pillow under your lower back to keep it arched. You can then adjust how much you bend your legs.

- ✔ A variation on the traditional missionary position is to lie on your front. You can then adjust your position to provide the most comfort for your back by placing a pillow under your chest or stomach or by propping yourself up on your elbows.

- ✔ You can modify the missionary position if you have one-sided spinal pain. Try lying on your back with one knee bent up and the other leg lying flat.

If you are a man with spinal pain, you can benefit from the missionary position in the following ways:

- ✔ A modified missionary position can be particularly useful if you have one-sided spinal pain. Place a pillow or two underneath your partner to raise her buttocks. You can then lie between her legs with one of your legs bent into a deep kneeling position, keeping your other leg straight behind you. The leg you bend and the leg you keep straight depend on the side of your spinal pain.

- ✔ A variation on the conventional missionary position (you probably had no idea of the versatility of this position!) is good if you find the standard position too painful. Ask your partner to lie on her back with one or two pillows underneath her back and buttocks. This position raises her enough to allow you to draw both knees into a kneeling position between her legs. You can then enter her in this position, putting minimal stress on your spine.

The female superior position

The female superior position is simply the woman on top. This position can be useful for both men and women with back pain.

For a man with spinal pain:

✔ This position allows you to keep your back comfortable and unstressed by straightening your knees or bending them upwards more, depending on what you find most comfortable.

✔ Try adjusting your position by using towels and pillows for support. This passive position allows you to protect your back while you enjoy intercourse.

✔ Your partner's movements can range from very gentle to more physically active. Keep her informed of your comfort level so she can adjust her movements in order to keep your pain at a minimum.

For a woman with spinal pain:

✔ This position allows you almost complete control over your physical movement. You can control the depth of penetration and speed of thrust, depending on your pain.

✔ Try resting your chest down on your partner's chest, which you may find more comfortable if rounding out your back reduces your pain.

✔ A variation on the standard female superior position, which also adds some creative variety to your experience, is to face away from your partner. Try this variation to see whether it provides you with more comfort.

Doggie style

Doggie style is the slang term for the position in which the man enters the woman from behind in the way most animals do. The woman is usually on all fours (on her hands and knees), with the man kneeling behind her. This position can be great for controlling spinal pain but may be a little hard on the man's knees if the surface isn't soft (of course, he can always go for knee pads).

For a woman with spinal pain:

✔ This position allows you to adjust the posture of your lower back, controlling your comfort level.

✔ You can position yourself with your torso more upright (by resting on pillows or the corner of the bed) or on your hands and knees on the bed.

For a man with spinal pain:

- ✔ This position can be comfortable because it allows you to keep your lower back rounded out.
- ✔ You can control the aggressiveness of your movements very effectively from this position in order to keep your pain at a minimum.

Side by side

Three side-by-side positions can be useful in managing spinal pain during sex: spooning, the T-bone, and the scissors position.

Spooning

Spooning is essentially a variation of the doggie style, but done sideways. In this position, the man enters the woman from behind, but the woman lies on her side rather than on her knees. Many couples find this position more physically relaxing than traditional doggie style.

For a man with spinal pain, the spooning position lets you control the position of your back during intercourse. You can adjust how you place your body next to your partner by bending your back slightly forwards or backwards, depending on what you find comfortable.

For a woman with spinal pain, spooning lets you control the position of your back by bending slightly forwards to bring your chest down towards your knees or by arching your back backwards and leaning towards your partner.

The T-bone

This position is good for both men and women with spinal pain. In the T-bone position, the woman lies on her back and the man lies beside her on his side, facing her. She bends both of her legs upward enough to allow him to bring his legs underneath hers. She then places her legs down over his. This position allows you and your partner to touch other body areas and have direct face-to-face communication.

For a woman with spinal pain:

- ✔ You are in a very relaxed and comfortable position.
- ✔ You can control the position of your back by how you position your legs.
- ✔ You can increase your comfort by placing a small towel or pillow under your lower back.

For a man with spinal pain:

- ✔ You control the position of your back during intercourse by how you place yourself next to your partner. You can lean forwards, closer to her, or away from her, depending on what you find most comfortable.

- ✔ You can control the aggressiveness of your movements while being in a position in which your entire body is supported by the bed – or lawn, or carpeting, or . . .

The scissors

In this position, the woman lies on her back and the man lies next to her on his side. The woman bends the leg closest to her partner; he brings his top leg forwards and places it under her bent leg. She then lowers her upper leg and rests it on top of his. Each partner has one leg bent and the other leg straight. (Keep rereading until it makes sense!) He can then enter her from the side.

This position can be quite comfortable if one or even both partners have general or one-sided back pain. This position is very relaxed for both partners and allows for face-to-face communication and touching.

Putting It All Together

We realise this chapter may seem overwhelming at first, but try to approach it in a fun and adventurous manner. We like to use the acronym GREAT SEX to summarise our advice for getting your relationship together – even with spinal pain:

- ✔ **Give it a try:** Begin by simply having a go at 'it'. 'It' may be anything in this chapter. Start out with whatever seems easiest for you and your partner, and then progress to other areas. Make communication one of the first 'it's to practise. Going through this chapter as a couple is an easy way to get started.

- ✔ **Romance and sensuality:** Don't forget that romance and sensuality are primary components of a good sexual relationship.

- ✔ **Express and communicate:** Expressing yourself and communicating in an open and non-threatening manner are important elements of a good relationship, particularly when it comes to sex and spinal pain.

- ✔ **Accentuate intimacy:** Remember to accentuate emotional and physical intimacy, especially when dealing with a spinal pain problem.

✔ **Time:** Make time and plan ahead for your romance, lovemaking, and sexual encounters. Don't count on spontaneity – and make sure that your sexual relationship happens.

✔ **Slow:** Go slowly when trying out the different things we discuss in this chapter. Proceed at a pace that keeps your pain at a minimum and avoids frustration, hostility, and defensiveness.

✔ **Explore variability:** As you work on your relationship, both emotionally and physically, make sure that you explore variations. Be creative and have fun!

✔ **Xcellent:** Okay, 'excellent' doesn't begin with an 'x'. However, we hope that after you and your partner work with this chapter a little, you can develop an excellent physical and emotional relationship regardless of your spinal pain.

Part VI
The Part of Tens

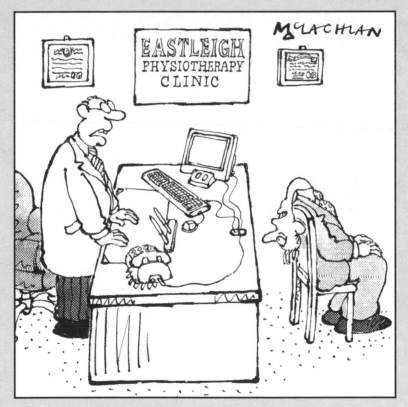

"I must say, Mr Pithycott,
you have the worst case of
whiplash I've ever seen."

In this part . . .

This is the fun part of the book. All *For Dummies* books include a Part of Tens, which features a few chapters that give you ten or so tips, ideas, or suggestions. These quick chapters condense information into little sound bytes that you can read on the run. Think of them as Top Ten lists with substance.

Chapter 20

Ten Common Questions about Back Pain

*R*emember the old saying 'The only silly question is the one you don't ask'? Well, as you deal with the medical community, you may feel that you should already know the answers to your questions – so much so that asking your doctor can be intimidating. In this chapter, we answer the ten most common questions that our patients ask about back pain. We hope that the answer to at least one of your own questions is here.

Can I Manage My Herniated Disc Without Surgery?

You can almost always manage your herniated disc successfully without surgery. Only a very small percentage of patients actually require surgery for a herniated disc (and we explain this in more detail in Chapter 3). Many studies show that patients with a herniated disc can recover well with non-surgical conservative management. In one study, 92 per cent of patients with disc herniations recovered without surgery. Many of these patients had large herniated discs that were compressing nerve roots. In another study, patients with disc herniations were treated surgically or non-surgically; after five years, the researchers found no difference between the two groups.

The symptoms of a herniated disc with nerve compression – back pain, buttock pain, and sciatica – often resolve spontaneously as the disc shrinks. Your body has a natural ability to heal and reabsorb disc herniations and return to a normal state.

Surgery may be appropriate for your disc herniation in some cases. If your neurological symptoms, such as weakness in your legs and decreased sensation, are getting progressively worse, your doctor may recommend surgery to prevent permanent neurological damage.

If you have bowel or bladder problems, seek medical advice immediately as you may have the cauda equina syndrome.

We discuss these issues further in Chapters 3 and 9.

What Kind of Practitioner Should I See for My Back Pain?

As we discuss in Chapter 4, many different health care professionals treat back and neck problems. You may find all the options quite confusing as you decide which type of medical practitioner to consult. Much of your choice depends upon your symptoms and history of back pain. For instance, if you have a long history of recurrent back pain, you probably already have a doctor you can consult when you have flare ups.

For acute back pain with no significant associated symptoms, such as bowel or bladder problems, debilitating pain down one or both legs, or severe throbbing pain that awakens you at night, see your GP, a chiropractor or osteopath (check out Chapter 11 for more on these), or a physiotherapist.

Your GP can give you a physical examination, rule out any serious problems, provide medication such as anti-inflammatories and painkillers (which we describe in Chapter 8), and recommend any appropriate limitations to your activity. Most GPs, however, don't provide specific instruction on back exercises.

An osteopath, chiropractor (both of which we describe in Chapter 11), or physiotherapist can provide initial treatment for your back pain. These practitioners cannot prescribe medication, but they may provide exercise guidelines.

Make sure that any practitioner you choose monitors you closely and focuses on gradually increasing your activities through strengthening and stretching. If your doctor primarily prescribes medications and recommends prolonged rest, consider consulting another doctor – research shows that this approach is likely to be ineffective and may actually make you worse.

If your back pain goes on for more than four to six weeks, you don't seem to be improving, and your activity level continues to be quite restricted, see a spinal specialist. Spinal specialists come in many guises. Doctors who specialise in spinal problems include orthopaedic surgeons, neurosurgeons, rheumatologists, and neurologists; they may work in a pain clinic. Choose a specialist who focuses on non-surgical conservative treatment of your back pain – rheumatologists often fill this role. See Chapter 4 for more information about the different specialists involved in back and neck pain. If you're interested in complementary treatments, you may want to find a spinal specialist who is comfortable working with alternative health care practitioners.

Why Do I Still Have Pain When My Imaging Scans Are Normal?

Many well-understood structural reasons for back pain may be applicable to your specific problem. However, in a large percentage of people with back pain, doctors find no specific identifiable diagnosis (see Chapter 3 for more on this). Your scans may be normal even though you still have discomfort, because your pain may come from parts of the body that current imaging technology can't identify. In fact, high-tech instruments may never be able to identify pain from, for example, inflammation, sprain, strain in the muscles or ligaments, or pain due to mental stress.

Therefore, imaging studies aren't the last word on diagnosing back pain. The results can also be difficult to interpret: Some people with no back pain have abnormal MRI scans whereas some people with back pain have normal MRI scans (see Chapter 7 for more on imaging studies). As we point out in Chapter 3, imaging studies and high-tech assessments are only part of a good evaluation of back pain.

The prognosis for a full recovery is extremely good, even if your doctors never find the exact cause of your back or neck pain. Treatments often work regardless of whether you know the exact cause of the pain.

What about Alternative Treatments for My Back Pain?

More and more people are pursuing alternative, or complementary, treatments for a variety of medical problems, including back and neck pain. Lots of complementary treatments are available for back and neck pain, and we review many of these in Chapters 10–13. Some of the more common complementary treatments for back pain include acupuncture, osteopathy, chiropractic, yoga, meditation, and bodywork.

Alternative treatment can complement conventional treatment for your back pain. Before pursuing any alternative treatments, however, ask your doctor to evaluate you to ensure that your pain doesn't stem from a serious problem that requires medical attention.

Look very carefully into any complementary medicine treatment, whoever provides the referral. To make sure that the alternative treatment you're receiving is safe, obtain answers to the following questions:

- ✔ Does this treatment involve any risk?
- ✔ How commonly is this treatment used for back pain?
- ✔ How long has this treatment been around?
- ✔ In what percentage of cases is this treatment successful for back pain?
- ✔ What are the potential side effects of this treatment?
- ✔ Can better or more orthodox treatments accomplish the same goal?
- ✔ How much, or how many sessions, of this treatment should I expect to undergo before I see results?
- ✔ How do you determine when and whether this treatment has been successful for my back pain?

Is My Diagnosis as Terrible as it Sounds?

As we mention in Chapter 3, doctors use a number of scary-sounding spinal diagnoses, but the reality of the condition may be nothing serious at all. Two such examples are *disc protrusion or bulge* and *degenerative disc disease*.

Disc bulges generally aren't a cause for concern and, in fact, are present in a high percentage of the population who don't even have any back or neck pain or other symptoms. Similarly, so-called arthritis of the spine and degenerative changes are often not associated with any back or neck pain. Spinal degeneration actually starts when you are about 20 years old and continues throughout your life. In the vast majority of cases, you can think of this condition as similar to other ageing processes, such as your hair turning grey.

When Should I Consider Surgery for My Back Pain?

Surgery is medically necessary to correct only a very few spinal problems. These conditions include severe nerve compression in the lower spine, spinal tumours, and some spinal infections. In all other situations, whether to have surgery is your choice: Making that decision can be very difficult. The guidelines we discuss in Chapter 9 and summarise in the following list can help you make a good decision:

- ✔ In most cases, consider surgery only after you've tried appropriate conservative treatment.

- ✔ Make sure that your surgeon has a very good idea of what's causing your pain and that he or she believes surgery can correct the problem.

- ✔ Be sure that your signs match your symptoms. In other words, that what is found and is therefore undisputable tallies with what you feel. Otherwise you may have an increased risk of surgical failure.

- ✔ Don't agree to exploratory surgery. Your surgeon should have a pretty good idea of what he or she is going to correct surgically. However, at times exploratory surgery is unavoidable.

- ✔ Try to eliminate psychological and emotional factors – such as depression, anxiety, and stress – that may get in the way of a good surgical response.

- ✔ Make sure that you have no other issues that may ruin your response to surgery, such as drug abuse or other medical problems.

- ✔ Consider surgery only if your back or neck pain is interfering with your quality of life to an unacceptable degree.

Can Stress and Emotion Cause My Back Pain?

Thoughts and emotions are part of any back pain problem. Take this issue seriously if you believe – or your doctor suggests – that stress is making your pain worse. Your thoughts and emotions, and the resulting stress you experience, have great power over the way you perceive pain: Stress and emotion can worsen any pain impulses coming from your back or neck.

Stress and emotion can even cause your pain. Doctors think that unconscious stress causes muscle tightness in your back. The resulting pain is similar to having a tension or stress headache in your back. In this situation, your pain originates entirely from emotional stress, and conventional medical treatments are unlikely to be effective until you address the emotional stress. For more information about stress-related back and neck pain, see Chapter 3.

How Can Pain Only in My Legs Be Related to My Back?

Think of a telephone line extending from the telephone exchange to your home. When the line just outside the terminal has a problem, you experience static on the line, even though you may be several miles away. Similarly, spinal nerves travel to your buttocks, down your legs, and all the way to your toes (see Chapter 2 for more on the parts of your spine). If something irritates the spinal nerves, you may experience pain anywhere along the nerve. So irritation of nerves in your lower spine can cause pain as far down as your feet and toes, even if you don't experience any pain in your back, buttocks, or upper legs.

What Makes Up a Good Medical Evaluation for Back Pain?

Before high-tech tests come into the picture, your medical evaluation needs to include a thorough history and physical examination (see Chapter 7 for more on physical examinations). The history and physical examination can usually categorise most back pain problems and determine whether you have a sprain or strain, a disc problem, or some other condition.

Your practitioner's physical examination may include specialised tests such as the straight-leg raise (asking you to lift each of your legs as you lie flat on your back to test disc problems); checking the sensations in your legs, ankles, and feet; checking your muscle strength, especially in your lower body; checking your reflexes; asking you to walk on the balls of your feet and then on your heels; and looking at your gait (how you walk).

After taking your history and doing a physical examination, your doctor may take an X-ray of your spine. Note that X-rays are generally not routine on your first visit to a doctor for back pain, although you can usually expect to have an X-ray if your pain started following a traumatic event, such as a car accident or a fall. In this case, your doctor uses the X-ray to look for fractures in your vertebrae.

Your doctor may also request blood and urine tests to assess other medical problems that may relate to your pain.

 Doctors reserve high-tech tests such as MRI and CT scans (which we describe in Chapter 7) for later on in your treatment, if necessary. These tests can help your doctor to confirm a diagnosis such as a herniated disc and to determine whether invasive conservative treatment such as nerve-block injections may be helpful. Some diagnostic tests, such as *myelography* and *discography* (both of which we discuss in Chapter 7), should be done only if you are considering spinal surgery.

Should 1 Continue Exercising if Doing So Worsens My Pain?

 The answer to this question really depends on your situation. First, if at any time your activities or exercise programme make your pain worse, consult your doctor. Given that proviso, we can then offer some general guidelines to answer this question.

In the acute or initial stages of your pain problem, let your pain be your guide. We recommend two days of bed rest – up to five days if necessary – after the onset of your pain, followed by a gradual increase in your activities (see Chapter 6 for more on bed rest and gentle exercise). As you increase your activities and add some exercises, stop or reduce if your pain worsens. Letting pain be your guide also applies to other spinal conditions that require a certain healing time, such as a spinal fracture and recovery from spinal fusion surgery.

If chronic pain causes *deconditioning* (you become physically weak from not using your muscles), expect to experience an increase in pain as you follow an exercise programme. This increase in pain is similar to the aches and pains you experience after a workout at the gym because you are using muscles that you haven't used for a while. In this case, you're experiencing 'good pain' because the pain indicates that you're getting stronger.

Even if you're receiving physical rehabilitation, consult your doctor if exercise causes your pain to worsen. Your doctor can check that your pain is part of your rehabilitation process and that you have no other problems or re-injuries.

Chapter 21

Ten Common Questions About Neck Pain

*O*ne of the services offered by BackCare (for full details, see Appendix B) is a helpline that responds to public enquiries about back and neck pain and associated problems. Over the years Myrad Kinloch has assessed much of this accumulated material. We are grateful to Myrad and BackCare for allowing us access to this information, which forms the basis of this chapter.

This chapter gives a clear picture of the main concerns of people with neck pain.

I've had Neck Pain for Years but my Doctor Says Nothing's Wrong and I Must Live With It. Is this True?

No! Such advice promotes helplessness, despair, and passivity and is contrary to current information and clinical practice – and yet this sort of advice is still quite common. Patients' dissatisfaction with the help they get for neck pain is widespread.

We urge you to try to get as much information from your practitioners as you can. We show you how to get the most out of consultations with your surgeon in Chapter 9, your complementary practitioners in Chapter 10, and your GP in Chapter 24. The more you know about and understand your condition, the more likely you are to be able to improve your situation.

I'm Going Out and Doing Less Because of My Neck Pain. Do You Have Any Advice?

You may be more concerned about the physical disability caused by your pain than you are by the pain itself. People with neck pain frequently describe themselves as 'housebound', say they 'can't go anywhere any more', or become concerned that they can't do household chores. They worry that as a consequence of not being able to sit or stand for long periods of time they may lose their jobs, or fear that they may become physically dependent on friends and family.

In Chapter 8 we describe pain programmes designed to address the problems we describe above. Unfortunately, although pain programmes are becoming more common, they still aren't common enough. If you don't have access to a pain programme, try applying their principles to your own situation.

Your attitude is important here – the more positive you are, the more likely you are to benefit. First, work out exactly what you are no longer doing – you may be surprised how much you've stopped doing. Then set yourself a gradually increasing list of targets to build up your activities. Start with what you know you can cope with, and then add to it bit by bit. Be prepared to put up with some pain. Remember that hurt doesn't necessarily mean harm.

Take heart that good results have been shown, time and again, to come from the efforts of following a pain programme. In Chapters 17–19, we give more detailed advice about these problems insofar as they relate to work, sport, and sex.

Why Have I had Three Different Diagnoses for my Neck Pain in as Many Weeks?

In most cases of neck pain, a specific diagnosis is not possible (we explain this in more detail in Chapter 3). However, practitioners still use hundreds of diagnostic labels for their patients with neck pain, such as 'slipped disc', 'trapped nerve', and 'cervical spondylosis'. Many different groups of people, including doctors and other health care practitioners, all with their own ideas and often with their own jargon, have contributed to the list of diagnostic labels. You are likely to receive different diagnoses from different practitioners for the same set of symptoms. These practitioners may offer widely differing, and sometimes contradictory, advice – a confusing and worrying situation to say the least.

A true specific diagnosis in a person with neck pain is very rare. And if a course of treatment isn't working for you, however confident your practitioner's diagnosis, be prepared to think again. In this field, what matters is what *works*.

Am I Ever Going to Find a Cure for My Neck Pain?

Understandably, many people with neck pain seek a cure for their condition. We detail many treatments in this book that can help with neck pain. If you still have neck pain but you haven't tried all the treatments we discuss in this book, we suggest you do so, as nobody can be sure of what may or may not work for you. If you've tried everything we mention in this book and still have pain, your chances of *complete* pain relief are relatively poor. However, you still have a good chance of reducing the level of disability caused by your pain. If your disability concerns you more than the actual pain, you can probably do something about that.

The search for a cure presents additional problems: You are looking for someone to give you a solution, but if that solution is to succeed, you need commitment, determination, and your own input.

What are the Pros and Cons of Neck Surgery?

We can't give a general answer to this question because each person is different. Remember that no surgeon embarks on a major procedure lightly. Planning your surgery is very important: List all your questions and anxieties before you see your surgeon. Your surgeon wants to discuss these issues with you because he or she doesn't want to operate on a patient who is confused or reluctant about surgery. Make sure that you are clear about everything your surgeon tells you. In Chapter 9, we give detailed information on how to communicate effectively with your surgeon.

I'm Worried that My Family Thinks I'm Malingering. What can I do?

You may worry about the effects of your pain and disability on both you and your family, leaving you feeling anxious, depressed, angry, or guilty. As we explain in Chapter 3, spinal pain has some inevitable psychological consequences. However, no evidence suggests that people with back and neck pain suffer any different psychological effects from people with other types of pain.

The common belief that a person with back or neck pain is malingering seems to be part of our culture, but no evidence exists to support this view. Unfortunately, many people admit to some anxiety when their doctor asks: 'Do you think you're putting this on?' or 'Do you think I or your family think that you're putting it on?'.

People with neck pain are often concerned that their family relationships may suffer as a result of their condition. Some people are concerned that they may become a 'burden' or that their family may withdraw their support and sympathy if the pain persists. Many people don't discuss their pain with their families – and yet discussing the matter is very important. After all, if the problem affects the whole family, it makes sense to face it as a family.

This brings us to the significance of psychological factors. Psychological factors are so important that in Chapter 13 we detail how to use psychological methods and techniques to help your situation.

Could My Headaches Originate in My Neck?

As many as one in three headaches may originate in the neck. If you have frequent headaches, ask your GP to examine your neck. Neck problems often cause one-sided headaches, which are commonly misdiagnosed as migraine. If your GP finds no clear cause of your headaches, consider consulting an osteopath or chiropractor (which we describe in Chapter 11), or an acupuncturist (for more on acupuncture, see Chapter 10), or physiotherapist. Alternatively, you may discuss with your GP having injections of local anaesthetic or steroids (which we talk about in Chapter 8).

An X-Ray Shows I Have Cervical Spondylosis. What does this mean?

After early middle age, cervical spondylosis is not only common but also universal. Cervical spondylosis is simply 'wear and tear'. Many doctors still believe that an X-ray finding of cervical spondylosis shows the cause of your neck pain, but this is absolutely not the case. After a certain age, everybody shows signs of cervical spondylosis but not everybody has neck pain. In fact, new episodes of neck pain tend to be fewer in later life, which is just one example of how damaging diagnostic 'labels' can be. A diagnosis of cervical spondylosis may make you feel that you're never going to get help for neck pain. But remember that one of the many treatments we outline in this book may well be effective. If your doctor puts your neck pain down to cervical spondylosis, ask for a specialist referral or consider using a complementary health care practitioner.

How Should I Deal With Whiplash Following a Car Accident?

Whiplash simply means a sprained neck. Most whiplash injuries settle down, heal, and cause no further trouble. However, a few whiplash injuries result in recurrent headaches, ringing in the ears, dizziness, and other symptoms more associated with ear, nose, and throat problems. Unfortunately, many doctors aren't aware of these symptoms of whiplash, which is a pity because the right treatment can be very helpful. Get medical advice immediately if you have a whiplash injury but sometimes problems may persist.

As a general guide, wait at least two weeks before consulting your GP if you have the symptoms described above: Within this period your neck may still heal of its own accord. Your GP may treat you or refer you to an osteopath, chiropractor, or another doctor with a specialist interest in whiplash injury. In particular, manipulation, acupuncture, and injections of local anaesthetic with or without steroids can be very helpful.

Can Neck Problems Cause Shoulder Pain?

Neck problems frequently cause shoulder pain. *Referred tenderness* is tenderness elicited at some distance from its true origin. This referred pain from the neck can produce physical signs that may indicate tennis elbow or *carpal tunnel syndrome* (a condition that causes pain and altered sensations in the hand) when in fact the symptoms are caused by problems in the spine. Pain between your shoulder blades often originates from your neck. If your practitioner doesn't consider this possibility, your treatment can prove unsatisfactory, because it may be targeted at the wrong place.

Chapter 22

Ten Steps to a Healthy Back and Neck

In This Chapter
▶ Staying healthy to help you avoid back and neck pain
▶ Planning for good health
▶ Incorporating healthy steps into your lifestyle

*O*ne of the best ways to treat back and neck pain is to prevent the pain from occurring in the first place whenever possible. You can help to achieve this aim by incorporating a few simple steps into your lifestyle that keep your back and neck healthy. This chapter contains ten common-sense methods that are good not only for your back and neck but also for your overall health.

Stay in Shape

The best way to keep your back and neck healthy is to stay physically fit. Try to take regular aerobic exercise. Some good overall conditioning activities that, done sensibly, are safe for your back and neck include brisk walking, swimming, certain types of aerobics (low impact or in the water), and cycling on a recumbent stationary bike (in which you sit in a semi-reclined position, with your back supported as you pedal). If you want to play sports, we recommend that you take part in an athletic activity that provides you with exercise and enjoyment. You're much more likely to follow through with an activity on a regular basis if you enjoy it. Regular aerobic exercise is good for your mental health too, because exercise relieves stress.

Do Your Back and Neck Exercises

Starting a home exercise programme for your back and neck can be a good way to keep your back and neck healthy. A good home exercise programme (we suggest one in Chapter 15) keeps your back, neck, and abdominal muscles in good shape. This type of programme used in conjunction with a cardiovascular or aerobic exercise programme is an excellent combination for a healthy back and neck.

Maintain Your Proper Body Weight

Being overweight can put stress on your body's structures, including your back. In particular, a pot-belly increases the stress on your lower back, setting you up for a back injury. Therefore, part of maintaining a healthy back involves eating healthily to try to maintain your proper body weight. Avoid the temptation to *crash diet* – starving yourself to get the weight off fast – which can be dangerous to your health and doesn't work over the long-term. To get help in setting up an effective weight-loss programme, consult a nutritionist or get involved with an organisation such as Weight Watchers (check your telephone directory for local numbers). Before starting any diet or exercise programme, consult your GP.

Watch Out for High-Risk Sports

We discuss a variety of different sports in connection with back and neck pain in Chapter 18. Certain sports involve a higher risk for spinal injuries than others. Apart from the obvious culprits – physically aggressive sports such as football – sports that require a lot of twisting can be risky. For instance, squash forces you to bend at the waist, twist, and hit the ball. This action can be stressful to your spine, especially if you don't warm up and stretch properly. Golf is another very twisty sport that can be hard on your spine – again, warming up and stretching properly before you play a round is important.

If you play sports that require lots of twisting, bending, or impact, take special care to follow a thorough warm-up routine. In many sports, especially golf and racquet games, you can take lessons with a professional to develop good techniques to minimise your risk of spinal injury.

Foster a Positive Attitude

Some research studies show that job dissatisfaction and other emotional variables can increase your risk of a back or neck injury with extended disability. Maintaining a positive attitude toward your job and home life can certainly help prevent a spinal pain problem. The converse is true too: If you already have a back or neck pain problem, maintaining a positive attitude in your work and home environments helps you recover more quickly. If you feel unable to maintain a positive attitude in these situations, talk with family and friends about options for solving the problems. Professional counselling can be helpful in this situation.

Lift and Move Properly

As we discuss in Chapter 14, lifting and moving objects properly is an important part of protecting your back and neck. When lifting an object, never bend over at the waist. Instead, bend at the knees, pull, and hold the object close to you, and lift from that position. Always look up before you lift to help put you in a proper lifting position.

Use common sense if you're thinking about trying to lift something too heavy. Stop and ask yourself whether lifting the object is worth the chance of an acute back or neck injury. If you think the object is too heavy for your back, get some help.

Don't Lift and Twist

Lifting an object and twisting at the same time is risky and may very well injure your back or neck. Turn your entire body rather than twisting your back as you lift a heavy object. Also, instead of throwing something heavy, try carrying or pushing it. Always stretch and warm up before any lifting or twisting activity such as playing sports. See Chapter 14 for more info on twisting and posture.

Don't Stand or Sit for Long Periods

If you need to stand for a long period of time, try changing your position frequently, and prop up one foot on a footstool. Leaning against something occasionally, such as a wall or column, can also be helpful. If you can predict when you may have to stand for a long time, plan to stretch, bend, or walk before your standing stint, or incorporate those activities into your regular breaks. Good supportive shoes are always helpful when you need to stand for long periods (see Chapter 14), as is a surface that absorbs some shock, such as a rubber mat or grass.

Long periods of sitting can also put a great deal of pressure on your spine. Driving is even worse because the road vibrations are transmitted to your spine. If you have to sit or drive for long periods, try to take a break at least once an hour to stretch, loosen up, and walk around.

Use a Good Chair

If you must sit for long periods of time, using a chair specially designed to put your back and neck in the most proper and healthy position can be very helpful (see Chapter 16). Many companies design ergonomically correct chairs for people whose jobs require them to sit for long periods, and some of these resources are listed in Appendix B. If you don't have a special chair, roll up a towel and place it behind your back for support as you sit. Propping your feet on a low footstool or a telephone book can also be helpful.

Avoid Carrying Heavy Luggage

To keep your spine healthy, avoid carrying heavy luggage when you travel. This advice is especially important when you travel regularly, for example as part of your job. Carrying heavy luggage on a shoulder strap can be awkward and stressful for your spine. Also, you're very likely to lift and twist heavy luggage as part of your travelling experience.

Your best bet is to get a trolley or luggage with wheels for long walks through airports and car parks. If no trolley is available and your suitcases don't have wheels, try to balance the weight of the load on each side of your body and take frequent breaks (see Chapter 14).

Chapter 23

(Almost) Ten Reasons to See a Doctor for Your Back or Neck Pain

- -

- -

*W*e very much believe that you can do a tremendous amount to manage your pain at home, on your own. In fact, we spend a good deal of time in Chapter 6 and elsewhere in this book explaining many self-care treatments. However, if you have certain symptoms, you need to see your doctor straight away. This chapter lists nine occasions when you need to head straight to a doctor, without passing Go.

You're Weak in the Legs or Feet

If you begin to experience weakness in one or both of your legs and/or feet, go to your hospital accident and emergency (A&E) department within 24 hours. With *foot-drop*, your foot becomes so weak that you have trouble pulling your toes up towards your head, causing your foot to drop and drag when you walk. Nerve compression in your spine may be the culprit (see the next section for more information).

You Can't Control Your Bowels or Bladder

Go to A&E immediately if you experience a loss of bowel or bladder control or any of the following symptoms:

- Loss of feeling during a bowel movement
- Inability to start or control your bowel movements
- Inability to start or control urination
- Loss of feeling in your groin or anal area
- Inability to get an erection (if you're male)

The *cauda equina syndrome* (which we describe in Chapter 9) may cause the symptoms we list above. This syndrome involves a compression or pressing on important nerves in your lower spine that supply function to your bowels and bladder and sensation to your groin and anal areas. Cauda equina syndrome usually requires immediate surgical treatment because permanent damage can occur if the nerves are compressed for too long.

Your Back or Neck Pain Awakens You

Your back or neck pain may wake you up every now and then. But *rest pain* – pain that consistently wakes you up – may rarely indicate a spinal infection or tumour. A bone scan or MRI scan can help diagnose these conditions (see Chapter 7 for more on these imaging studies). People with weakened immune systems may be at greater risk of getting spinal infection or a tumour.

The constant throbbing or aching pain that occurs with a tumour or spinal infection may be quite severe throughout the day and worsen with rest. The pain may be markedly different from the back or neck pain that occasionally awakens you at night. Although a tumour or spinal infection is not quite as severe a medical emergency as cauda equina, still see your GP with a view to being referred to a spinal specialist quickly if you notice symptoms of rest pain (see Chapter 9 for more on cauda equina).

You Have New Symptoms or Excruciating Pain

Ask your GP to refer you to a spinal specialist as soon as possible or go to A&E if you have excruciating pain that is unbearable. 'Unbearable' is a subjective description but is usually defined as pain that makes you go to hospital or see a doctor because you just can't stand it.

- ✔ If your pain kicks in when your GP's surgery is closed or you don't have a spinal specialist, go straight to A&E.
- ✔ If you have a spinal specialist or you have been seeing your GP about your pain, ask that person for guidance on what to do. If you're unsuccessful, go to A&E.

Call your GP or specialist if you experience any new symptoms associated with your back or neck pain, such as bowel or bladder problems, foot-drop or weakness, and radiating pain, numbness, tingling, or shooting pains in your legs.

You Have a Serious Accident

If your pain starts after, or is worsened by, a serious accident such as a bad fall, call a doctor. Try to contact your GP or spinal specialist first, but if your pain is unbearable and your doctor unavailable, go straight to A&E.

Although most people with back or neck pain don't require an imaging study such as an X-ray or CT scan (which we describe in Chapter 7), if you've had an accident your doctor may need to use imaging tests to check for vertebral fractures (for more on these, see Chapter 3).

A vertebral fracture is not usually a serious problem and requires only limited rest, time to heal, and appropriate treatment, such as wearing a brace, restricting your activities, and/or using certain medicines. After the fracture heals, your spine usually returns to functioning normally and painlessly. However, a small percentage of spinal fractures are unstable and require surgery to repair them (as we explain in Chapter 9).

You Want to Pursue Complementary Treatments

We believe that the most powerful treatment approach is to combine both conventional and complementary medicine in an appropriate manner. Part III gives the low-down on some of the most popular forms of complementary medicine.

If you decide to seek complementary treatment for your pain, ask your doctor to evaluate you first (see Chapter 10 for tips on how to work with your doctor and a complementary practitioner in conjunction). A medical evaluation ensures that your back or neck pain isn't due to a serious condition. After your medical evaluation rules out any significant problems, you can pursue your complementary medicine treatments without worry.

You Need More than an Aspirin for Your Pain

You can use a number of home remedies to treat your back or neck pain, including limited bed rest, ice and heat, over-the-counter anti-inflammatory and painkilling medicines, and mild exercise. (See Chapter 6 for more information on self-treatments.) If these approaches don't work adequately, see your GP. Your GP can suggest other treatments such as physiotherapy and stronger medicines. (In Chapter 8, we give more information about the medical treatment of back and neck pain.)

You're not Seeing any Improvement

Conservative treatments for your back and neck pain include home remedies and more formal treatment such as physiotherapy. Specialists in back and neck pain often prescribe a course of four to six weeks of physiotherapy and then follow you up again when you're reassessed to see what your course of physio has achieved.

Physiotherapy can aggravate your pain initially as you increase your activity. After a few weeks, however, you begin to feel some relief from your symptoms. If you don't notice any improvement, see your doctor before ending the physiotherapy. If the physiotherapy doesn't seem to be helping, or is hurting, consult your GP. Your GP may suggest changing the physiotherapy approach or adding other treatments, such as medication, nerve blocks, or complementary approaches (which we describe in Chapter 8) to make the physiotherapy more effective.

Your Medication Isn't Working

If you're taking medication for your back or neck pain, pay attention to how you feel. If one of the follow situations arises, see your GP.

- **You experience side effects to the medication:** Your doctor may want to alter your dosage or switch you to another medication. (We describe some of the different medications used for back and neck pain in Chapter 8.)

  Herbs are medicines too. Always tell your doctor when you're combining herbal and prescription medicines. If you experience side effects, your doctor may need to consider the possibility of interactions between the various medications you're taking.

- **You're using drugs to self-medicate your pain:** Self-medicating in this case includes taking more medication than your doctor has prescribed, drinking alcohol to treat your back or neck pain, taking someone else's medication, and using other drugs such as marijuana or opiates to manage your pain.

Chapter 24

(Almost) Ten Tips for Working Successfully with Your Doctor

. . . .

In This Chapter

▶ Practising assertive communication

▶ Planning a visit to your doctor in advance

▶ Maintaining a positive attitude

▶ Exploring other sources of information

. . . .

Surveys show that generally most people are satisfied with the care they get from their doctors (throughout this chapter the term doctor means a medically qualified practitioner, whether GP or spinal specialist). Unfortunately, good care doesn't always translate into good communication. Patients commonly make the following complaints about their doctors:

✔ My doctor doesn't spend enough time with me.

✔ My doctor isn't friendly.

✔ My doctor doesn't answer questions openly.

✔ My doctor doesn't explain problems clearly.

✔ My doctor doesn't treat me with respect.

As busy professionals, doctors are sometimes lacking in the active communication department. But you can help too. The ability to work with your treatment providers effectively is a critical part of enhancing your response to treatment. The tips in this chapter show you how to communicate with your doctor while preserving the quality of the overall relationship. By following these techniques, you and your doctor can work together to create the best possible treatment programme for you.

Identify Your Communication Style

Your personal communication style can have a great impact on your relationship with your doctor. Research shows that people tend to use one of four different types of communication. You may notice that you tend to use one style of communication in one type of situation and a completely different style in other interactions.

- ✔ **Non-assertive or submissive behaviour:** This communication style is giving in to another person's preferences and discounting your own rights and needs. When you're chronically non-assertive, you may feel the need to please others around you, and be afraid that people aren't going to like you when you express your own desires. At the same time, you may feel guilty or resentful that your rights are being 'violated', but in reality no one knows how you feel. People around you may not even realise that you're non-assertive or submissive because you never express your needs.

- ✔ **Aggressive behaviour:** This communication style involves expressing your wants and desires in a hostile or attacking way. Aggressive people are typically insensitive to the rights and feelings of others around them and use coercion and intimidation to get what they want. People targeted with aggressive communication respond in one of two ways: They leave the situation or they become defensive and fight back.

  Being aggressive when seeking treatment for your back or neck pain can be disastrous. An aggressive attitude towards your practitioners can cause them to withdraw from you or counter-attack in a similarly aggressive manner.

- ✔ **Passive-aggressive behaviour:** This communication style is a means of expressing anger in a passive manner. Passive-aggressive people tend to express hostile urges or anger in a sullen, disgruntled way that obstructs the wishes of others. Passive-aggressive behaviour is designed to frustrate others by such actions as postponing decisions, constantly raising objections, or taking ineffective action. Expressing anger in a passive-aggressive way is a very ineffective means of communication that usually leaves your needs unmet and others around you frustrated.

- ✔ **Assertive communication:** This communication style is the expression of how you feel or what you want while respecting the rights of others. Assertive communication is simple and direct without attacking, manipulating, or dismissing those around you. See the next section for tips on communicating assertively.

Become an Assertive Communicator

You can develop your ability to communicate in an assertive fashion. Try following these guidelines to help you be assertive with your doctor:

- ✔ **Use assertive non-verbal behaviour:** Your body language goes above and beyond your verbal expression. Assertive behaviour includes such things as establishing eye contact, keeping your head up, standing straight, maintaining an *open posture* (facing the other person, with your head up and arms uncrossed), and staying calm.

- ✔ **Keep your request simple:** An assertive request is simple, direct, and straightforward. Ask for only one thing at a time: A multitude of requests can be quite confusing for your doctor. Easy-to-understand sentences such as 'I'd like more information about my treatment programme' and 'I'd like more information about how to obtain a second opinion' are effective and assertive communications.

- ✔ **Be specific:** Before you see your doctor, determine your wants, needs, and feelings so that you can express them in a specific fashion. Avoid vague requests such as 'I'd like to get more help from your surgery staff regarding your recommendations', which your doctor may not interpret correctly. Instead, opt for the more effective 'I'd appreciate your staff's help with setting up my appointment for the MRI, and getting me information about pain control.'

- ✔ **Use 'I' statements:** People have a tendency to tell others what they want them to do by using 'you statements' such as 'You need to help me out more.' To the person listening, these statements may feel threatening, which puts the receiver on the defensive. Instead, use 'I statements', which frame your request in terms of your own needs. 'I'd like to understand my treatment plan better' elicits a totally different response from 'You're not giving me enough information about my treatment.'

- ✔ **Avoid the temptation to address personality flaws and concentrate on behaviours instead:** You may be tempted to say 'I know that as a doctor you're very impatient, but can you explain this test to me again?' Your doctor responds to your needs much more favourably when you say 'I'd like you to explain this test to me again so that I understand my treatment better.'

- ✔ **Don't apologise for your request:** If you're a non-assertive communicator, you may have trouble believing that your request deserves a response. This feeling surfaces in your statements: 'I'm really sorry to ask, but can you, if possible, explain the test results again?' With an apologetic approach, your request is often ignored. Instead, go with a more assertive 'I'd appreciate you explaining the test results again.'

  ✔ **Don't make demands:** Assertive communication involves making a request of another person or setting a limit by saying 'No'. In both cases, always communicate in a way that respects the rights and dignity of the other person.

Plan Your Consultation in Advance

Before you see your doctor, think about what you want to get out of this particular consultation and then make a list of your questions and concerns in a simple and straightforward format. Be realistic about the number of questions you can ask during any given consultation. Although you may feel that you should be able to spend as much time with your doctor as you like, and ask as many questions as you want, time pressures mean that this simply isn't possible. Your doctor needs to balance the time available for all his or her patients throughout the day.

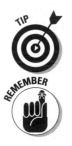

As you look over your list of concerns and questions, try to summarise them into five or so main questions, to allow adequate time for discussion. Write down the questions and take them with you to ensure that you remember what to ask your practitioner.

Communicating your goals at the outset can help the consultation go smoothly. For instance, you may start out your visit by telling your doctor that you have five questions or concerns that you want to discuss.

Prepare Your Medical Fact Sheet

Writing up a *medical fact sheet* – a written summary of your important medical information – can help you get the best treatment and avoid dangerous or harmful mistakes. Most hospitals send you a fact sheet to fill out before your initial specialist consultation. Check to make sure that the doctor's fact sheet contains at least the following information and then add any information not included. Otherwise, compile your own fact sheet, which needs to be concise and neat and include at least the following information:

  ✔ Your name, address, telephone numbers, emergency contacts, and any special problems or disabilities you have.

  ✔ Current medical conditions, with brief explanations.

  ✔ Previous treatments and your responses to them.

  ✔ Previous medical tests and the results of them.

   ✔ Past medical conditions, with brief explanations and dates.

   ✔ Surgical history, with dates and outcomes.

   ✔ Current medications, with dosages and side effects.

   ✔ Allergic reactions to medications.

   ✔ Other practitioners involved in your medical care, with contact details and the conditions they are treating.

After you prepare your medical fact sheet, take a copy to each of your health care professionals. Providing this information helps them to co-ordinate your treatments and do a better job overall.

Check Your Attitude

Your attitude about your medical consultation can affect the outcome greatly. For instance, when you're angry because you're in pain or you don't like going to a doctor, you're likely to be aggressive. Although some doctors are more understanding than others about your pain and the associated irritability, most doctors meet aggressiveness with defensiveness or counter-aggressiveness: Neither situation leads to a pleasant, productive consultation.

Another way to keep your cool is to bring along something to do as you wait for the doctor to see you. Your attitude can go from pleasant to sour when you're left in the waiting room with magazines from the early 1960s. Take an interesting piece of reading material – this book, maybe? – or something else to keep yourself pleasantly occupied – such as knitting or a pocket computer game.

Many people believe that doctors don't value their patients' time but demand that patients respect theirs. Although some doctors certainly have such an attitude, most keep their patients waiting only when uncontrollable circumstances arise, such as an urgent phone call, an emergency patient visit, or an operation that goes on longer than expected. Unfortunately, in the world of health care, these unforeseen problems happen more frequently than in other lines of work.

Allow the Doctor to Ask Questions First

Your doctor needs to gather a great deal of information in a relatively short period of time, so let him or her ask questions first. After that, you can ask for any information not covered or for clarification of anything unclear. Even though waiting to give your doctor information that you think is important can be difficult, resist the urge to go into the visit with a prepared monologue because you may end up giving the doctor information not relevant to your diagnosis and treatment. Your doctor may open with questions about how you're getting on and what symptoms you're experiencing. Answering these opening questions is your opportunity to tell your doctor what's happening. The doctor has to gather certain information in order to formulate a treatment plan and assess your progress. After he or she obtains that information, you can express your specific questions and concerns.

Make Sure that You Understand the Conclusions

Summarise any conclusions you and your doctor come to at the end of the consultation. If you're uncertain about any instructions or guidelines, address these before you leave. You may want to take notes during the consultation, but avoid getting so focused on recording every detail that you don't pay attention to what your doctor is saying. If you don't understand a recommendation – especially relating to medication – be sure to ask for clarification.

Bring a Friend

Bringing a friend or relative is an effective way to get the most out of your consultation – especially when you're facing an important medical decision or gathering information from a specialist.

- Your friend's presence has a calming and relaxing effect, allowing you to focus better on the important stuff.

- You're less likely to feel intimidated with someone else with you.

- Your companion can bring up questions or concerns and help you recall the discussion with the doctor. When you and your friend don't agree on what was heard, you can raise these questions with your doctor on the next visit.

- Your friend can act as a reality check on how the consultation went.

Using the suggestions we present in this chapter, you may want to develop an overall strategy for your doctor's consultation with your friend or family member beforehand.

Explore Other Sources of Information

You may be able to get further information about your back or neck pain from sources other than your doctor. For instance, your doctor may mention a certain diagnosis or treatment approach but not go into much detail due to time constraints. You may be able to find more information by reading books about the problem or procedure, searching the Internet, and joining self-help groups. The resources in Appendix B can be a good place to start searching out more information.

Scrutinise carefully the source and content of the information you obtain, especially from the Internet. Information on the Internet is completely unregulated and often invalid. Many patients have been unduly frightened by information they find concerning their diagnosis and/or treatment plan. Appendix B has several good Web sites for collecting more medical information.

Part VII
Appendixes

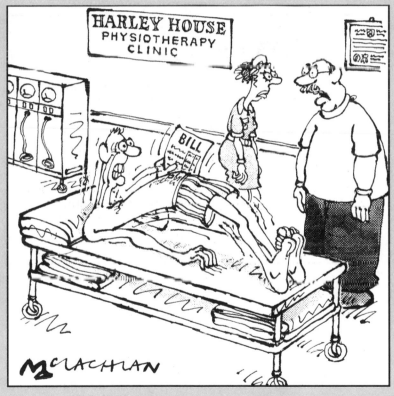

"I'd just got him _completely_ relaxed & then you go & give him the bill!"

In this part . . .

Small but perfectly formed, these Appendixes are bursting at the seams with useful information. Appendix A is an at-a-glance glossary of back and neck pain terms used in this book. Don't know your CAT scan from your MRI? Appendix A can sort you out.

Appendix B provides essential information about product providers and helpful organisations, all back and neck pain related. From trusted yoga practitioners to hypnotherapists specialising in pain control, use Appendix B as a springboard to finding more help for your condition.

Appendix A

Glossary

● ●

*T*his glossary defines many of the most important – and often most confusing – terms that you encounter reading this book or working with your back and neck pain practitioner. Cross-referenced terms are in ***bold italics***.

Acupoints: *Acupuncture* points throughout the body that correspond to specific organs. Acupoints are found along the ***meridia***.

Acupuncture: Ancient Chinese medicine approach in which small needles that pierce the skin are placed at specific body locations (***acupoints***) to cause healing or other benefits, for example pain relief.

Acute back or neck pain: Back or neck pain that has a rapid onset, severe symptoms, and short duration. In contrast to chronic back or neck pain, acute back or neck pain is sometimes defined as continuing for less than three months.

Anaesthetic: Any substance that causes a loss of sensation or feeling, especially pain.

Analgesic: Pain-relieving substance.

Ankylosing spondylitis: Inflammatory disease of the spine. More common in men than women.

Annulus fibrosis: Tough fibrous outer portion of the intervertebral disc.

Anterior: Towards the front or forward part of the body or an organ.

Anti-anxiety medications: Medications used for the relief of anxiety. Also termed **anxiolytics**.

Antidepressants: Medications that provide relief from depression. In much lower doses than those used to treat depression, they can also provide pain relief and help with sleep.

Anti-inflammatories: Substances that decrease the inflammatory response of tissues and reduce swelling and pain. Examples include ibuprofen, diclofenac, naproxen, and aspirin.

Arachnoiditis: Inflammatory condition of the spinal **arachnoid** – the connective tissue around the spinal cord. Arachnoid literally means like a cobweb, which describes how the structure appears on imaging studies.

Arthritis: Inflammation and irritation of the joints that often includes swelling and pain. A normal effect of ageing that responds well to exercise.

Biofeedback: Treatment approach in which a physical response or symptom such as muscle tension, heart rate, sweat-gland activity, or blood pressure is electronically measured and fed back to you so you can discover how to bring it under voluntary control.

Bodywork: Term referring to therapies such as massage, deep-tissue manipulation, movement awareness, and energy balancing.

Bone scan: Scan or *X-ray* taken after injection of a radioactive dye, which is allowed to concentrate in the skeleton. The primary use of a bone scan is to diagnose a fracture, infection, tumour, or *arthritis* of the bones. Any area of increased concentration of the dye is significant.

Bulging disc: Intravertebral disc that sticks out only slightly from its normal space without breaking through the *annulus fibrosis*. The disc may or may not cause any symptoms. See also *protrusion* and *sequestration* and contrast with *extrusion*.

Bursitis: Inflammation of the *bursa* – a sac-like cavity filled with lubricating fluid and located within a joint.

Cervical spine: Seven vertebrae that comprise the neck area of the spine.

Chemonucleosis: Treatment in which a chemical is injected into the disc in order to dissolve the part of it thought to cause symptoms. Because of possible severe side effects, this treatment is rarely used.

Chi: See *Qi*.

Chiropractic: Treatment approach that focuses on the relationship of the spinal column, muscles, and skeleton. Spinal *manipulation* and other treatment techniques are utilised, such as a variety of soft tissue techniques to help mobilise joints.

Chronic back or neck pain: Back or neck pain that persists for a long time – usually more than three months. Also defined as pain beyond the point of tissue healing. Commonly termed **chronic benign back or neck pain**.

Coccydynia: Pain in the *coccyx* or tail bone area.

Coccyx: Small bone at the end of the sacrum; the tail bone.

Cognitive/cognition: Thought; related to thinking.

Conservative treatment: Non-surgical treatment that doesn't cause irreversible changes.

CT or CAT scan: Computerised *X-ray* visual recording of sections or slices of your body. Short for computerised (axial) tomography.

Deconditioning syndrome: Generally refers to the negative consequences of resting your body too much due to spinal pain. Also termed **disuse syndrome**.

Degeneration: Gradual tissue change resulting in lower or less active function. Commonly used to describe ageing changes in the spinal *discs*.

Degenerative disc disease: Condition in which *disc* degeneration, usually at several spinal levels, causes pain.

Disc (intervertebral): Cartilage tissue comprising 80 per cent water and sitting between two vertebrae. A disc has two main parts: the outer ring (*annulus fibrosis*) and the inner ring (*nucleus pulposus*). Discs separate the spinal vertebrae and act as shock absorbers.

Disc degeneration: Progressive, normal process during which *discs* lose water and shrink in size. Disc degeneration may or may not cause symptoms and commonly occurs as part of the normal ageing process. This term is used interchangeably – but inaccurately – with *degenerative disc disease*.

Disc narrowing: Occurs when a *disc* degenerates to the point of reducing the distance between two adjoining vertebrae. This is a normal part of the ageing process.

Discectomy: Surgical removal of all or part of a *disc* (usually in the case of a *herniated disc*).

Discography: Test in which radioactive dye is injected into a *disc* to see whether the injection of the dye causes the patient to experience his or her usual pain, thereby confirming the disc as a source of pain. The recorded result of this test is called a *discogram*.

Dura: Tough, protective, outermost membrane surrounding the spinal cord and brain.

Electrodiagnostic studies: Any test of nerve function in which electricity is used. Nerve conduction studies and electromyography (EMG) are the most common examples.

Endorphins: Chemicals produced in your brain, which act as natural painkillers.

Enzymes: Complex proteins that are produced by living cells and catalyse specific biochemical reactions.

Epidural injection: Injection of an anaesthetic or other substance into the *epidural space*.

Epidural space: Area just outside the *dura* in the spinal canal.

Ergonomics: Study of how you use your body in situations such as work, sports, and other settings. The interaction between the body and the environment.

Extension: Bending the spine backwards.

Extrusion: Displacement of a portion of the *disc* through the *annulus* into the spinal canal. Contrast with *bulging disc*, *protrusion*, and *sequestration*.

Facet joints: Paired joints that connect the *posterior* (towards the back) aspects of the *vertebrae*.

Failed back surgery syndrome: Chronic back-pain syndrome that develops after one or more unsuccessful spinal operations.

Fascia: Fibrous membrane covering, supporting, and separating muscles. Unites skin with the underlying tissue.

Fibromyalgia: Clinical syndrome defined by specific points of muscle tenderness, sleep disturbance, diffuse pain, and fatigue.

Foramen: Natural passage or opening in a bone or membrane; often an opening through which a nerve passes.

Fusion: Process of 'melting' together. Spinal fusion is an operation in which bone grafts are placed in between two or more *vertebrae*, with the goal of having them grow together. Spinal fusion reduces the mobility or movement in that part of the spine.

Gate-control theory of pain: Theory that postulates that spinal nerve gates can open, allowing more pain messages to reach the brain, and close, allowing fewer pain messages to reach the brain, due to a variety of factors. These gates cause the perception of more or less pain in your brain.

Hemilaminectomy: Surgical removal of a *lamina* on only one side.

Herbal therapy: Ancient treatment approach that includes tablets or liquids loaded with plant extracts used for treating illness.

Herniated disc: Extrusion or herniation of the nucleus of a *disc* through the *annulus fibrosis*. If the herniated disc material irritates or compresses a nerve, the result can be symptoms such as pain, weakness, or numbness down the leg.

Hydrotherapy: Any therapy or treatment that uses water.

Hypnotherapy: Treatment to induce a trance-like state to foster healing; supposedly bypasses the conscious mind, which may be impeding progress or causing illness. Hypnotherapy can boost your positive thoughts and aid recovery.

Hypochondriasis: Irrational fear of presumed illness and a preoccupation with the body.

Idiopathic back or neck pain: Back or neck pain that doesn't have a well-known or identifiable cause. Investigations indicate that most spinal pain is idiopathic, even though practitioners give some type of diagnosis.

Imaging studies: General term referring to tests that give an image of a body part or structure such as *CT scan*, *magnetic resonance imaging (MRI)*, and *X-ray*.

Impotence: Loss of a male's ability to maintain an erection to the point of ejaculation.

Invasive treatment: Any procedure that includes penetrating the skin. This type of treatment is differentiated from non-invasive *conservative treatment*.

Kinesiologist: Practitioner trained in the anatomy and mechanics of movement.

Kinesophobia: Irrational fear of movement; often part of the development of *deconditioning syndrome* and *chronic back pain*.

Lamina: Part of the *vertebra* just behind the spinal canal.

Laminectomy: Operation to remove part of the *lamina*. Usually done to relieve pressure on the spinal cord and the nerves coming from it.

Laminotomy: Surgical creation of an opening in the *lamina*.

Lesion: Any injury, pain, or damage.

Ligament: Band of fibrous tissue that connects bones or cartilage or supports and strengthens joints.

Lumbar spine: The region including five *vertebrae* that make up the lower back area of the spine.

Lumbar stenosis: Narrowing (stenosis) of the spinal canal in the *lumbar spine*.

Lumbosacral sprain/strain: Ambiguous term for injury to the muscles, ligaments, or tendons of the back.

Magnetic resonance imaging (MRI): Commonly used imaging technique that uses a strong magnetic field rather than *X-rays* and reveals anatomical structures in great detail.

Magnetic therapy: Use of magnetic fields to treat various disorders, including back and neck pain.

Manipulation: Use of pressure or force by a practitioner such as a chiropractor, osteopath, or physiotherapist to cause movement of the bones of the spine. The cracking noises that are often heard are the result of gases released from the joints. Also termed **adjustment** or **joint mobilisation**.

Meridia: In Eastern tradition, the major energy pathways throughout the body along which *qi* runs.

Modality: Most commonly refers to the **passive modalities** in which you are the passive receiver of a physiotherapy treatment such as massage, heat, cold, or ultrasound.

Muscle spasm: Involuntary contraction or tightening of muscles.

Musculoskeletal system: Skeleton and its muscles.

Myelography (or CT-myelography): *X-ray* and/or *CT scan* done after injection of a contrast or radioactive dye into the spinal canal. Used for better viewing of body structures. The side effects (most notably severe headache) of this procedure have decreased dramatically following the creation of water-soluble dyes. This test should be done only when you are considering surgery.

Myositis: Inflammation of the muscles.

Nerve root: Part of the nerve that leaves the spinal canal, goes through the *foramen*, and extends just beyond the *vertebrae*. Several nerve roots come together to form larger nerves such as the sciatic nerve.

Neurological: Pertaining to the study of diseases of the nervous system.

Neurologist: Consultant doctor who has advanced training in problems of the nervous system. Neurologists use non-surgical treatment approaches.

Neuromuscular: Pertains to both the nerves and the muscles.

Neurosurgeon: Consultant surgeon who specialises in treating problems of the nervous system.

Neurotransmitters: Substances that transmit nerve impulses to the brain.

Nucleus pulposus: Inner part or centre of a *disc*.

Objective: In medicine, a symptom or condition that is perceptible to other people as well as the patient – the opposite of *subjective* findings. For example, *X-ray* results are objective findings but pain is subjective.

Opiates: Medications that contain opium or any of its derivatives; narcotics.

Organic: Explicable by physical causes or related to being physical. In outdated medical jargon, pain was defined as organic or functional (refers to a psychological or emotional basis). Currently, this distinction is not useful and shouldn't be used.

Orthopaedic surgeon: Consultant surgeon specialising in the surgical treatment of the *musculoskeletal system*.

Osteopathy: Treatment approach that focuses on the relationship between the spinal column, muscles, and skeleton. Spinal manipulation and other treatments are used.

Osteoporosis: Weakening of the bones as they lose some of their density.

Pain clinic: Multidisciplinary treatment centre that uses a variety of specialists to evaluate and treat pain in a highly co-ordinated and structured fashion. Pain programmes usually emphasise you taking personal responsibility for getting well.

Paracetamol: A non-narcotic pain reliever that doesn't have anti-inflammatory properties. Less irritating to the stomach and intestinal tract than anti-inflammatory medicines.

Pedicle: Bony part of the *vertebrae* that connects it to *posterior* structures. In *fusion* surgery, the site of placement for pedicle screws.

Physiotherapist: Clinician trained in the treatment of *musculoskeletal* problems. Treatment is based on exercise and other physical interventions.

Pinched nerve: Non-medical term for compression of a nerve.

Podiatrist: Practitioner with training in the evaluation and treatment of problems of the feet.

Posterior: Situated towards the back.

Protrusion: Distinct bulge in the *annulus fibrosis* due to displaced *disc* material. See also *bulging disc* and *sequestration* and contrast with *extrusion*.

Pseudoarthrosis: Condition in which a *fusion* has been attempted but inadequate healing of the bone grafts in between the *vertebrae* result in incomplete union.

Psychiatrist: Consultant doctor who specialises in the practice of *psychiatry*, the branch of medicine concerned with the study and treatment of disorders of the mind.

Psychological: Pertaining to emotions, mental processes, thoughts, and human behaviours.

Psychologist: Practitioner trained in the evaluation and treatment of problems related to mental processes, emotions, and behaviours. To treat back or neck pain, a psychologist needs specialised training in pain management.

Psychosomatic: Describes a physical condition that results from, or is made worse by, psychological factors. Also termed **psycho-physiological**. These conditions are often – incorrectly – considered to be imaginary problems; however, actual physical changes occur due to non-physical forces. See *stress-related back pain*.

Qi: In complementary medicine, the vital life energy that runs throughout the body (also spelled **chi**).

Range of motion: Physiological range of joint movement in several different directions.

Recurrent acute back or neck pain: Episodes of back or neck pain of varying duration and separated by relatively pain-free periods. Possibly the most common type of back or neck pain.

Rheumatologist: Consultant doctor who specialises in arthritic problems.

Ruptured disc: See *herniated disc*.

Sacroiliac (SI) joint: Joint between the sacrum and pelvis. Two SI joints exist, one on each side of the sacrum.

Sacrum: Thick triangular bone situated at the lower end of the spinal column, where the column joins the pelvis.

Sciatica: Pain in the distribution of the sciatic nerve, down the legs.

Scoliosis: Abnormal curve of the spine. Often very mild and usually doesn't cause symptoms. In severe cases, the condition can be treated with bracing or surgery.

Sedatives: Medication used primarily to induce sleep. Also referred to as **hypnotics**.

Sequestration: Complete displacement of part of a *disc* into the spinal canal with no connection to the remaining disc; also termed a **free fragment**. Contrast with *bulging disc*, *protrusion*, and *extrusion*.

Specificity theory of pain: States that a one-to-one relationship exists between pain and the amount of tissue damage. Proposed by Descartes hundreds of years ago, but now known to be inaccurate.

Spinal canal: 'Tube' through which the spinal cord passes. Formed by the opening at the back of each vertebra as they stack upon one another.

Spinal stenosis: Abnormal narrowing of the spinal canal. Classified as **developmental** (genetic), **congenital** (present from birth), or **acquired** (developed after birth). Acquired stenosis is the most common form due to degenerative changes in the spine.

Spinous processes: Bony bumps on the *vertebrae* to which muscles and *ligaments* attach.

Spondylitis: Inflammation of the *vertebrae*, usually due to normal wear-and-tear changes associated with ageing. Rarely a cause of back pain.

Spondylolisthesis: Slipping forward of an individual *vertebra* over the vertebra below it.

Spondylosis: Degenerative changes of the spine, including the *vertebrae*, the *discs*, and the *facet joints*.

Sprain: Injury in which some of the fibres of a supporting *ligament* are ruptured.

Strain: Over-exercising, overstretching, or overexertion.

Stress-related back or neck pain: Back or neck pain thought to be caused and maintained primarily by emotional and psychological issues.

Subjective: Pertaining to medical findings that are a symptom or condition perceptible only to the patient. Subjective needs to be contrasted with *objective*. Pain is a subjective symptom.

Tendons: Tough cord or band of dense white fibrous connective tissue that attaches a muscle to some other body part.

Thoracic spine: The 12 vertebrae that comprise the middle part of the back. The most stable part of the spine due to the attachment of the ribs. Rarely a source of back pain.

Traction: Treatment in which pressure is applied to the spine in order to pull the *vertebrae* away from one another.

Transcutaneous nerve stimulation (TENS): Treatment in which low levels of electricity are applied to areas of pain through electrodes placed on the skin for pain relief.

Ultrasound: Use of sound waves to generate heat below the surface of the skin to aid the healing process.

Vertebra: Bone of the spine. Each vertebra has three parts: the vertebral body, the transverse process, and the spinous process. The word *vertebrae* is the plural form of vertebra.

X-ray: Form of electromagnetic radiation. A tissue or organ that is dense, such as bone, absorbs more X-radiation than the surrounding tissue. This difference in density produces a relative transparency or picture on the film.

Appendix B

Resources for Additional Information

· ·

*T*his appendix lists some organisations and Web sites as a good starting point for collecting information relating to your back or neck pain. These resources can provide you with more information about your back and help you find out about different practitioners and centres that deal with back and neck pain and related conditions.

Organisations

The organisations in this section can provide you with more information about back and neck pain. These resources can help you find a specific type of spinal pain specialist and treatment method. Although making such a list exhaustive is impossible, these organisations can probably provide you with many other resources in their specific area.

Acupuncture

British Acupuncture Council, 63 Jeddo Road, London, W12 9HQ. Tel: 020-8735-0400. Web site: www.acupuncture.org.uk

British Medical Acupuncture Society, BMAS House, 3 Winnington Court, Northwich, Cheshire, CW8 1AQ. Tel: 01606-786-782. Web site: www.medical-acupuncture.co.uk

Alexander technique

Society of Teachers of the Alexander Technique, First Floor, Linton House, 39–51 Highgate Road, London, NW5 1RS. Tel: 0845-230-7828. Web site: www.alexandertechnique.uk.com

Alternative and complementary medicine (general)

Complementary Medical Association, The Meridian, 142a Greenwich High Road, London, SE10 8NW. Web site: www.the-cma.org.uk

Federation for Integrated Medicine, 12 Chillingworth Road, London, N7 8QJ.

The Centre for Complementary and Integrated Medicine, 56 Bedford Place, Southampton, Hampshire, SO15 2DT. Tel: 02380–334-752. Web site: www.complemed.co.uk

Institute for Complementary Medicine, PO Box 194, London, SE16 7QZ. Tel: 020-7237-5165. Web site: www.i-c-m.org.uk

Ankylosing spondylitis

National Ankylosing Spondylitis Society (NASS), Parkshort House, 5 Kew Road, Richmond, Surrey, TW9 2PR. Tel: 020-8334-7026. Web site: www.nass.co.uk

Arthritis

Arthritis Care, 18 Stephenson Way, London, NW1 2HD. Tel: 0845-600-6868 (24hr) or 020-7380-6500. Web site: www.arthritiscare.org.uk

Arthritis Research Campaign, Copeman House, St Mary's Court, St Mary's Gate, Chesterfield, Derbyshire, S41 7TD. Tel: 0870-850-5000. Web site: www.arc.org.uk

Aromatherapy

International Federation of Professional Aromatherapists, 82 Ashby Road, Hinkley, Leicestershire, LE10 1SN. Tel: 01455-637-987. Web site: www.ifparoma.org

Aromatherapy Consortium, PO Box 6522, Desborough, Kettering, Northants, NN14 2YX. Tel: 0870-774-3477. Web site: www.aromatherapy-regulation.org.uk

Bodywork

Light Touch Therapy, Tel: 01837-840-718. Web site: www.lightouch.co.uk

Association of Systematic Kinesiology, 47 Sedlescombe Road South, East Sussex, TN38 0TB. Tel: 0845-020-0383. Web site: www.systematic-kinesiology.co.uk

Feldenkrais Guild UK, 13 Camellia House, Idonia Street, London, SE8 4LZ. Tel: 07000-785-506. Web site: www.feldenkrais.co.uk

Chiropractic

British Chiropractic Association, 59 Castle Street, Reading, Berkshire, RG1 7SN. Tel: 0118-950-5950. Web site: www.chiropractic-uk.co.uk

General Chiropractic Council, 44 Wicklow Street, London, WC1X 9HL. Tel: 020-7713-5155. Web site: www.gcc-uk.org

Consumer information and protection

Consumer Protection Service, County Hall, Beverley, East Riding of Yorkshire, HU7 9BA. Tel: 08454-040-506. Web site: www.eastriding.gov.uk/environment/consumerprotection

Drugs, medications, and products

Medicines and Healthcare Products Regulatory Agency, 10-2 Market Towers, 1 Nine Elms Lane, London, SW8 5NQ. Tel: 020-7084-2000. Web site: www.mhra.gov.uk

Fibromyalgia

Fibromyalgia Association UK, PO Box 206, Stourbridge, West Midlands, DY9 8YL. Web site: www.fibromyalgia-associationuk.org

Homeopathy

Homeopathic Medical Association, 7 Darnley Road, Gravesend, Kent, DA11 0RU. Tel: 01474-560-336. Web site: www.the-hma.org

Society of Homeopaths, 11 Brookfield, Duncan Close, Moulton Park, Northampton, NN3 6WL. Tel: 0845-450-6611. Web site: www.homeopathy-soh.org

Hypnosis and hypnotherapy

British Society of Medical and Dental Hypnosis, 28 Dale Park Gardens, Cookridge, Leeds, LS16 7PT. Tel: 07000-560-309. Web site: www.bsmdh.org

General Hypnotherapy Register, PO Box 204, Lymington, SO41 6WP. Tel: 01590-683-770. Web site: www.general-hypnotherapy-register.com

National Council for Hypnotherapy, PO Box 421, Charwelton, Daventry, NN11 1AS. Tel: 0800-952-0545. Web site: www.hypnotherapists.org.uk

Massage therapy

General Council for Massage Therapy, 27 Old Gloucester Street, London, WC1N 3XX. Tel: 0870-850-4452. Web site: www.gcmt.org.uk

Meditation

Himalayan Institute of Great Britain, 21 Humes Avenue, London, W7 2LJ. Tel: 0208-567-8889. Web site: www.himalayaninstitute.org.uk

Mental health

Mental Health Care, Institute of Psychiatry, King's College London, De Crespigny Park, London, SE5 8AF. Tel: 020-7836-5454. Web site: www.mentalhealthcare.org.uk

Mind (National Association for Mental Health), 15–19 Broadway Stratford, London, E15 4BQ. Tel: 020-8519-2122. Web site: www.mind.org.uk

Naturopathy

General Council and Register of Naturopaths, Goswell House, 2 Goswell Road, Street, Somerset, BA16 0JG. Tel: 08707-456-984. Web site: www. naturopathy.org.uk

Nutrition

British Nutrition Foundation, High Holborn House, 52–54 High Holborn, London, WC1V 6RQ. Tel: 020-7404-6504. Web site: www.nutrition.org.uk

Food Standards Agency, Aviation House, 125 Kingsway, London, WC2B 6NH. Tel: 020-7276-8000. Web site: www.food.gov.uk

Osteopathy

British Osteopathic Association, 3 Park Terrace, Manor Road, Luton, LU1 3HN. Tel: 01582-488-455. Web site: www.osteopathy.org

British School of Osteopathy, 275 Borough High Street, London, SE1 1JE. Tel: 020-7407-0222. Web site: www.bso.ac.uk

European School of Osteopathy, 104 Tonbridge Road, Maidstone, Kent, ME16 8SL. Tel: 01622-685-989. Web site: www.eso.ac.uk

General Osteopathic Council, 176 Tower Bridge Road, London, SE1 3LU. Tel: 020-7357-6655. Web site: www.osteopathy.org.uk

Pain (general)

Pain Relief Foundation, Clinical Sciences Centre, University Hospital Aintree, Lower Lane, Liverpool, L9 7AL. Tel: 0151-529-5820. Web site: www. painrelieffoundation.org.uk

British Pain Society, Third Floor, Churchill House, 35 Red Lion Square, London, WC1R 4SG. Tel: 020-7269-7840. Web site: www.britishpainsociety.org

Reflexology

British Reflexology Association, Monks Orchard, Whitbourne, Worcester, WR6 5RB. Tel: 01886-821-207. Web site: www.britreflex.co.uk

Support groups

Arachnoiditis Trust, 20 Hopefield Chase, Rothwell, Leeds, LS26 0XX. Tel: 0113-288-0121. Web site: www.arachnoiditistrust.org

BackCare, 16 Elmtree Road, Teddington, Middlesex, TW11 8ST. Tel: 020-8977-5474. Web site: www.backcare-helpline.org

Disabled Living Foundation, 380–384 Harrow Road, London, W9 2HU. Tel: 020-7289-6111. Web site: www.dlf.org.uk

National Association for the Relief of Paget's Disease, 323 Manchester Road, Walkden, Worsley, Manchester, M28 3HH. Tel: 0161-799-4646. Web site: www.paget.org.uk

National Osteoporosis Society, Camerton, Radstock, Bath, BA2 0PJ. Tel: 0845-130-3076. Web site: www.nos.org.uk

Pain Concern, PO Box 13256, Haddington, EH41 4YD. Tel: 01227-712183. Web site: www.painconcern.org.uk

Scoliosis Association UK, 2 Ivebury Court, 323–327 Latimer Road, London, W10 6RA. Tel: 020-8964-5343. Web site: www.sauk.org.uk

Spinal Injuries Association, SIA House, 2 Trueman Place, Oldbrook, Milton Keynes, MK6 2HH. Tel: 0800-980-0501. Web site: www.spinal.co.uk

Surgery

British Orthopaedic Association, 35–43 Lincoln's Inn Fields, London, WC2A 3PE. Tel: 020-7405-6507. Web site: www.boa.ac.uk

Yoga

British Wheel of Yoga, 25 Jermyn Street, Sleaford, Lincolnshire, NG34 7RU. Tel: 01529-306-581. Web site: www.bwy.org.uk

Yoga Biomedical Trust, 90–92 Pentonville Road, London, N1 9HS. Tel: 020-7689-3040. Web site: www.yogatherapy.org

Product Resources

You may want to check out the following places for products that can help relieve your back pain:

Anatomia (Back 2), 28 Wigmore Street, London, W1U 2RN. Tel: 020-7935-0351. Web site: www.back2.co.uk

Advanced Seating Designs, Unit H, Field Way, Metropolitan Park, Greenford, Middlesex, UB6 8UN. Web site: www.asd.co.uk

The Back Care Warehouse, 2a Tower Road, Worthing, West Sussex, BN11 1DP. Tel: 01903-204-140. Web site: www.thebackcarewarehouse.co.uk

The Back Shop, 14 New Cavendish Street, London, W1G 8UW. Tel: 020-7935-9120. Web site www.thebackshop.co.uk

Bodycare, EZL Marketing Limited, Unit 23A, North Tyne Industrial Estate, Benton, Newcastle-upon-Tyne, NE12 9SZ. Tel: 0191-266-8887. Web site: www.ezl.co.uk

Putnums Back Support Products, Eastern Wood Road, Langage Industrial Estate, Plympton, Devon, PL7 5ET. Tel: 01752-345-678. Web site: www.putnams.co.uk

Index

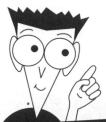

FOR DUMMIES®

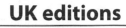

Do Anything. Just Add Dummies

HOME

UK editions

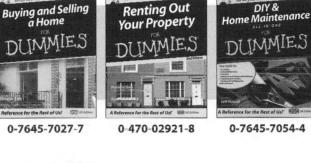

0-7645-7027-7 **0-470-02921-8** **0-7645-7054-4**

PERSONAL FINANCE

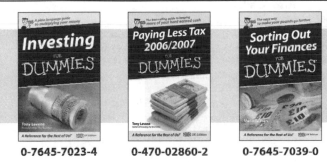

0-7645-7023-4 **0-470-02860-2** **0-7645-7039-0**

BUSINESS

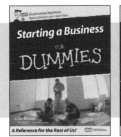
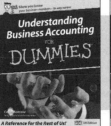

0-7645-7018-8 **0-7645-7025-0** **0-7645-7026-9**

Answering Tough Interview
Questions For Dummies
(0-470-01903-4)

Arthritis For Dummies
(0-470-02582-4)

Being the Best Man
For Dummies
(0-470-02657-X)

British History
For Dummies
(0-470-03536-6)

Building Confidence
For Dummies
(0-470-01669-8)

Buying a Home on a Budget
For Dummies
(0-7645-7035-8)

Buying a Property in Eastern
Europe For Dummies
(0-7645-7047-1)

Children's Health
For Dummies
(0-470-02735-5)

Cognitive Behavioural Therapy
For Dummies
(0-470-01838-0)

CVs For Dummies
(0-7645-7017-X)

Diabetes For Dummies
(0-7645-7019-6)

Divorce For Dummies
(0-7645-7030-7)

eBay.co.uk For Dummies
(0-7645-7059-5)

European History
For Dummies
(0-7645-7060-9)

Gardening For Dummies
(0-470-01843-7)

Genealogy Online
For Dummies
(0-7645-7061-7)

Golf For Dummies
(0-470-01811-9)

Hypnotherapy For Dummies
(0-470-01930-1)

Irish History For Dummies
(0-7645-7040-4)

Marketing For Dummies
(0-7645-7056-0)

Neuro-linguistic Programming
For Dummies
(0-7645-7028-5)

Nutrition For Dummies
(0-7645-7058-7)

Parenting For Dummies
(0-470-02714-2)

Pregnancy For Dummies
(0-7645-7042-0)

Retiring Wealthy For Dummies
(0-470-02632-4)

Rugby Union For Dummies
(0-470-03537-4)

Small Business Employment
Law For Dummies
(0-7645-7052-8)

Starting a Business on
eBay.co.uk For Dummies
(0-470-02666-9)

Su Doku For Dummies
(0-470-01892-5)

The GL Diet For Dummies
(0-470-02753-3)

Thyroid For Dummies
(0-470-03172-7)

UK Law and Your Rights
For Dummies
(0-470-02796-7)

Wills, Probate and Inheritance
Tax For Dummies
(0-7645-7055-2)

Winning on Betfair
For Dummies
(0-470-02856-4)

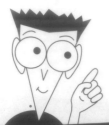
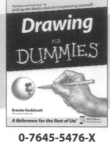
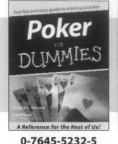
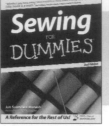
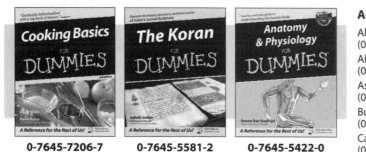
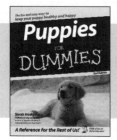
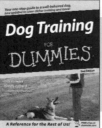
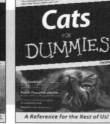

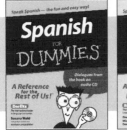

FOR DUMMIES®

The easy way to get more done and have more fun

LANGUAGES

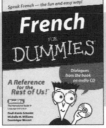

Speak Spanish — the fun and easy way!

Spanish FOR DUMMIES®

A Reference for the Rest of Us!

0-7645-5194-9

Speak French — the fun and easy way!

French FOR DUMMIES®

A Reference for the Rest of Us!

0-7645-5193-0

Start speaking Italian in no time with this fun and easy guide

Italian FOR DUMMIES®

A Reference for the Rest of Us!

0-7645-5196-5

Also available:

Chinese For Dummies
(0-471-78897-X)

Chinese Phrases
For Dummies
(0-7645-8477-4)

French Phrases For Dummies
(0-7645-7202-4)

German For Dummies
(0-7645-5195-7)

Italian Phrases For Dummies
(0-7645-7203-2)

Japanese For Dummies
(0-7645-5429-8)

Latin For Dummies
(0-7645-5431-X)

Spanish Phrases
For Dummies
(0-7645-7204-0)

Spanish Verbs For Dummies
(0-471-76872-3)

Hebrew For Dummies
(0-7645-5489-1)

MUSIC AND FILM

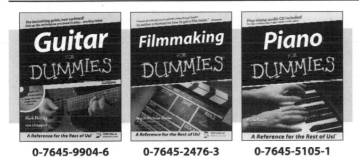

The bestselling guide, now updated! Pick up the techniques you need to play — starting today

Guitar FOR DUMMIES®

A Reference for the Rest of Us!

0-7645-9904-6

Filmmaking FOR DUMMIES®

A Reference for the Rest of Us!

0-7645-2476-3

Play-along audio CD included!

Piano FOR DUMMIES®

A Reference for the Rest of Us!

0-7645-5105-1

Also available:

Bass Guitar For Dummies
(0-7645-2487-9)

Blues For Dummies
(0-7645-5080-2)

Classical Music For Dummies
(0-7645-5009-8)

Drums For Dummies
(0-471-79411-2)

Jazz For Dummies
(0-471-76844-8)

Opera For Dummies
(0-7645-5010-1)

Rock Guitar For Dummies
(0-7645-5356-9)

Screenwriting For Dummies
(0-7645-5486-7)

Songwriting For Dummies
(0-7645-5404-2)

Singing For Dummies
(0-7645-2475-5)

HEALTH, SPORTS & FITNESS

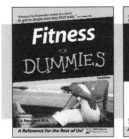

"Fitness For Dummies makes it a cinch to get in shape and stay that way."

Fitness FOR DUMMIES®

A Reference for the Rest of Us!

0-7645-7851-0

The fun and easy way to tone up and slim down with today's hottest exercise aids

Exercise Balls FOR DUMMIES®

A Reference for the Rest of Us!

0-7645-5623-1

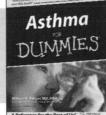

"Every person with asthma or allergies should own this book!"

Asthma FOR DUMMIES®

A Reference for the Rest of Us!

0-7645-4233-8

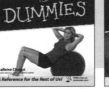

Also available:

Controlling Cholesterol
For Dummies
(0-7645-5440-9)

Dieting For Dummies
(0-7645-4149-8)

High Blood Pressure
For Dummies
(0-7645-5424-7)

Martial Arts For Dummies
(0-7645-5358-5)

Menopause For Dummies
(0-7645-5458-1)

Power Yoga For Dummies
(0-7645-5342-9)

Weight Training
For Dummies
(0-471-76845-6)

Yoga For Dummies
(0-7645-5117-5)

Available wherever books are sold. For more information or to order direct go to www.wiley.com or call 0800 243407 (Non UK call +44 1243 843296)

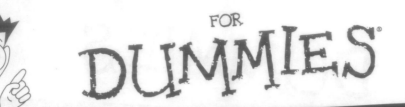
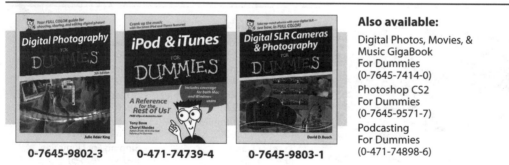
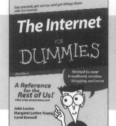
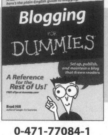
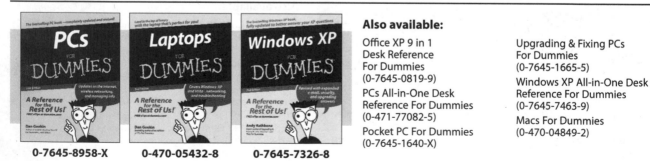

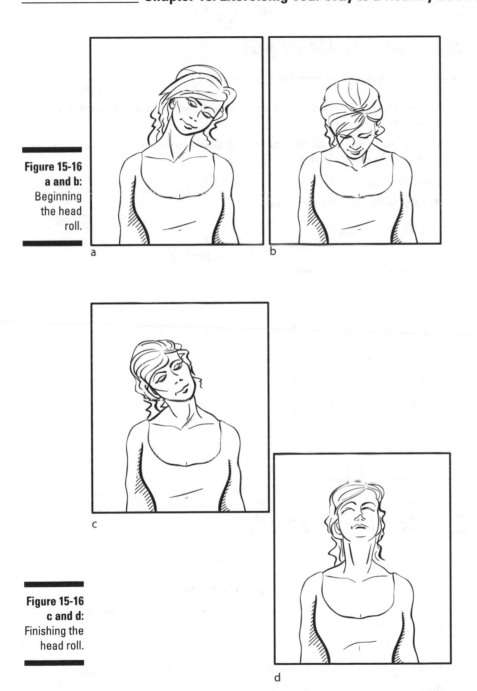

Figure 15-16 a and b: Beginning the head roll.

a

b

c

Figure 15-16 c and d: Finishing the head roll.

d